Habits

A Simple Framework for Transforming Your Habits

(*Wellness Habits Reprogram Your Mind for Aesthetic Goals*)

Mark Owens

Published By **Jordan Levy**

Mark Owens

All Rights Reserved

Habits: A Simple Framework for Transforming Your Habits (Wellness Habits Reprogram Your Mind for Aesthetic Goals)

ISBN 978-1-7772796-8-4

No part of this guidebook shall be reproduced in any form without permission in writing from the publisher except in the case of brief quotations embodied in critical articles or reviews.

Legal & Disclaimer

The information contained in this book is not designed to replace or take the place of any form of medicine or professional medical advice. The information in this book has been provided for educational & entertainment purposes only.

The information contained in this book has been compiled from sources deemed reliable, and it is accurate to the best of the Author's knowledge; however, the Author cannot guarantee its accuracy and validity and cannot be held liable for any errors or omissions. Changes are periodically made to this book. You must consult your doctor or get professional medical advice before using any of the suggested remedies, techniques, or information in this book.

Upon using the information contained in this book, you agree to hold harmless the Author from and against any damages, costs, and expenses, including any legal fees potentially resulting from the application of any of the information provided by this guide. This disclaimer applies to any damages or injury caused by the use and application, whether directly or indirectly, of any advice or information presented, whether for breach of contract, tort, negligence, personal injury, criminal intent, or under any other cause of action.

You agree to accept all risks of using the information presented inside this book. You need to consult a professional medical practitioner in order to ensure you are both able and healthy enough to participate in this program.

Table Of Contents

Chapter 1: Power Of Habits 1

Chapter 2: How External Factors Affect Habits 31

Chapter 3: Neglect And Customary Habit 48

Chapter 4: How To Be Proactive 81

Chapter 5: 11 Habits Of Not Viable To Withstand People 101

Chapter 6: How To Become Your Own Hero 108

Chapter 7: The Extraordinary Feasible Manner To Begin A New Addiction 119

Chapter 8: The Thriller Mastery Of Self Control 140

Chapter 9: Time Management 143

Chapter 10: Cultivating Adaptability 150

Chapter 11: The Role Of Consistency In Skill Development 163

Chapter 12: Gratitude And Positivity.... 174

Chapter 1: Power Of Habits

STEPS BY STEP GUIDES TO START NEW HABITS AND BREAK THE BAD ONES

Different techniques are needed to shape new behavior and damage horrible ones.

Developing new conduct may be a existence changing way with profound consequences. Starting a new addiction consists of careful thought and analysis, regardless of whether or not your cause is to stay a higher lifestyle, increase productiveness, or look at a cuttingedge functionality. We'll test the critical steps to successfully starting and keeping a modernday addiction in this bankruptcy.

Understanding the Cycle of Habits

Habits have a critical and frequently unconscious issue in the complex net of human behavior. The addiction loop, a neural pattern that affects our conduct frequently with out our facts, is at the coronary heart of addiction formation. Cue, Routine, Reward are the three vital components of this loop.

1. The Triggered Signal or Cue: cue can be either inner or outdoor, reason behavior to upward push up. External cues can include the time of day, a place, or the presence of certain people. Emotional states like pressure, boredom, or enthusiasm might probable feature internal cues. The first step in developing a contemporary day dependancy is privy to your cues. To start the dependancy loop, you may deliberately assemble a reason with the beneficial resource of identifying what reasons your selected movement.

CUE AND TRIGGER PURPOSE The Clever Cues are the subliminal cues that cause the start of a dependancy in our minds.

These cues may be divided into some of firstrate instructions, along with:

Timebased totally absolutely Cues: A timeprimarily based definitely cue is an event that takes location regularly in time or at a given component in time and reasons a positive movement. It serves as a temporal reminder that, counting on the immediately of the occasion, motivates you to participate in a specific motion.

As an instance, putting an alarm to remind you to go for a quick stroll each hour can function a timeprimarily based absolutely reason to sell ordinary movement all sooner or later of the day. Another instance is brushing your tooth earlier than bed; getting equipped for bed acts as a cue that the addiction have to be finished at a specific time. Timebased definitely really indicators are a fulfillment at forming conduct because of the fact they establish a sample and hyperlink the numerous favored conduct and a particular time.

They make it much less hard at the manner to create a ordinary timetable for sporting out particular responsibilities, growing the chance that the dependancy turns into embedded for your each day ordinary.

Locationbased totally definitely Cues: A areaprimarily based surely cue is a specific environment or placing that motives a certain behavior or dependancy. It's a visible or environmental cue that motivates you to perform a specific motion. Locationbased symptoms are often hired in behavior and behavior exchange techniques.

If you hold your gym apparel next for your mattress, as an instance, seeing them first component within the morning can act as a cause to encourage you to exercise. Similar to this, having a pitcher of water for your desk will characteristic a reminder to drink plenty of water in the end of the day.

Emotional Cues: A sure emotional nation or temper that reasons a selected conduct or reaction is referred to as a "emotional cue." Emotionalbased signs are feelings or emotions that cause the onset of a dependancy, whether they will be real or terrible, within the context of addiction formation or behavior amendment.

As an instance, stress ought to likely act as an emotional cue that units off the addiction of pressure eating. Similar to feeling bored, scrolling through social media as a kind of enjoyment may be caused through emotional cues.

Psychological Cues: These cues are often linked to cognitive capabilities and, relying on our highbrow nation, would probably have an impact on the manner we behave.

An character might in all likelihood, for instance, have a psychologyprimarily based cue that, when they're concerned, makes them want to exercising deep respiratory as a coping method. Another instance will be to apply encouraging terms as a cue to enhance confidence earlier than a tough hobby.

Since they act as the starter for the addiction loop, it is critical to realise the cues that motive your favored conduct.

Cue Association: Our brains increase stable connections amongst cues and sporting activities over time. This explains why unique cues will usually cause a specific conduct. For example, if you have a tendency of grabbing for a snack even as you are harassed out (an emotional cue), your thoughts will recommend a hunger for that snack the moment anxiety devices in. Understanding the ones hyperlinks permits you to take manage and deliberately choose an opportunity response.

2. The Routine: The Action itself

"Routine" comes subsequent within the addiction loop after the "cue" and springs earlier than the "praise." When you reply to the cue, you absolutely act or behave in a fine way. As a part of the bigger addiction loop, the habitual is the recurring conduct you carry out.

The ordinary is the path of movement you have a look at to address the purpose that the cue gives. It's the movement you over and over engage in for the duration of time.

For example, if your cue is feeling compelled, your everyday can be going for a hint stroll to clean your head, and your praise might be feeling a whole lot less traumatic and more focused.

The ordinary is essential considering that it's miles the movement you need to turn into a addiction. The neural pathways on your brain are reinforced by way of manner of constantly doing the habitual in response to the sign, which over time allows the dependancy come to be more automatic and ingrained. The sample will become much less tough and more convenient to perform over the years, and the addiction loop gets stronger.

Effect of Routine: The impact of the regular is to set up a reliable behavioral sample that is in step with your preferred goals or outcomes.

The exercise turns into a whole lot less hard worklarge to complete while it's miles repeated increasingly. This is because of the fact the mind can support and form new connections among neurons, which make it less tough to initiate the habit in response to the stimulus.

As the exercising is repeated, it has some of effects:

Efficiency: With repeated use, the exercise turns into easier to finish and more powerful, requiring less aware attempt. In reaction to the cause, your mind starts offevolved offevolved to assume the normal, which makes your actions seem predictable.

Consistency: The addiction loop motivates you to carry out the everyday continuously, which enables you make bigger an extendedlasting addiction.

Automaticity: With sufficient practice, the recurring will become embedded on your conduct, allowing you to carry out the motion absolutely with out questioning. As the system is carried out greater often, it calls for lots lots less attempt to carry out. This is so that the addiction may be started out out more results in response to the stimulus because the mind has the capability to create new and improve present neural connections. Repeating the workout gives some of benefits:

Positive Results: If your ordinary is normal along with your goals, regular of completion of the routine can also result in rewards or favorable outcomes, that may improve the addiction loop.

Since the normal is the movement you want to turn into a addiction, it's far an important a part of the dependancy loop. You ought to make it much less complicated to perform the behavior over time with the useful resource of strengthening the neural connections associated with the dependancy by way of manner of the usage of focused on performing the routine in response to the sign

three. The Reward (The Benefit): The praise is the favorable forestall give up result or gain you bought from executing this machine. Rewards can be fabric (like a tasty address) or intangible (like a experience of fulfillment). Dopamine, a neurotransmitter linked to pleasure and reinforcement, is launched with the useful resource of your mind even as it receives the praise.

This dopamine release makes it a good deal less complex so that you can repeat the addiction inside the future with the aid of way of strengthening the link most of the cue and the behavior.

With a reward, each addiction loop is completed. Rewards are a hit outcomes that satiate cravings or goals, strengthening the addiction loop and growing the risk that you could repeat the hobby inside the future. A sensation of serenity, less tension, or a sense of fulfillment is probably the advantages of our meditation instance. The first rate comments loop this is produced by way of the use of manner of the mind's affiliation of the praise with the conduct develops the dependancy over the years.

On the possibility facet, extrinsic incentives involve outside reinforcement, in conjunction with compliments from others or fabric advantages like a cope with or a financial incentive. Both kinds of rewards help human beings create conduct, however intrinsic rewards are plenty extra effective at maintaining longlasting behaviors.

Dopamine and the Brain: Dopamine is a neurotransmitter that the thoughts releases in response to worthwhile and exciting sports. Your mind strengthens the addiction loop whilst you've got interaction in a routine that effects in a terrific praise. You may also moreover apprehend the mind's integrated mechanisms and use them on your advantage if you apprehend how dopamine functions in dependancy formation.

The Effect of Rewards in a Chain

Rewards characteristic the dependancy loop's supply of motivation. For new behavior to be installation and sustained, it's far essential to understand the psychology of incentives.

Postponed Reward a few conduct pay off you later; they call for persistence and staying power. One of the maximum essential abilties in addiction formation is the capacity to postpone gratification, or the capability to reject briefterm income in pick out out of lengthyterm advantages. Developing now not on time gratification strengthens your strength of will and equips you to stay together together with your addiction even on the same time as you do not see any on the spot blessings.

By incorporating the ones insights into your approach for growing new behavior, you'll be higher able to create effective cues and take advantage of the psychology of incentives. You can create a strategic plan that increases your probabilities of achievement by means of way of identifying the triggers that cause your behaviors and comprehending the function that rewards play in strengthening conduct. Keep in thoughts that the complex interaction among cues, triggers, and rewards holds the essential trouble to unlocking the general capability of addiction development as you circulate beforehand on your addictionbuilding adventure. We'll discover sensible techniques for setting up addictionfriendly environment, handling resistance, and growing the consistency required to generate longlasting satisfactory alternate inside the components that observe.

CASE STUDY

Let's take a look at a few realglobal case studies of individuals who correctly started out new behavior to better understand the electricity of the dependancy loop:

Let's preserve in thoughts the example of Vanessa, a earnings earner who used a behavior loop to beautify her financial state of affairs and attain her dreams.

Evelyn aimed to growth her budget and start saving for her exceptional tour. She used a behavioral loop to try this. She commenced thru manner of creating a price range outlining her profits, expenses, and economic financial savings targets. She examined her finances every month and saved song of her spending to make certain she stayed on direction.

Evelyn computerized her monetary financial savings through putting in a direct rate into a delegated financial financial savings account as a part of her conduct loop. She modified into able to commonly make contributions to her vacation fund as a give up cease end result, heading off the temptation to divert the finances.

Evelyn also superior the exercise of keeping up along with her private economic training. To acquire information approximately cash control, funding possibilities, and strategies for achieving her dreams, she studied books, went to seminars, and found monetary specialists.

Evelyn's disciplined method eventually produced consequences. The quantity she had saved for her best excursion multiplied slowly as she watched it technique its aim. Her motivation to live together with her addiction loop or even locate greater strategies to keep money got here from the firstclass feedback she acquired from looking her fulfillment.

The money for Evelyn's quality revel in subsequently came collectively. She have turn out to be capable of fulfill her excursion ambition due to the fact to her regular efforts and conscientious spending practices, which additionally located her on the road to superior economic balance and health.

Evelyn stepped forward her monetary scenario, took the adventure she had expected, and found out crucial schooling approximately smart cash control through her conduct loop. Her revel in demonstrates the rate of forming reliable exercises for salaried those who need to benefit financial dreams.

Let's have a study every other instance: Meet Brian, a driven guy with a preference to decorate his health and shed pounds.

He intentionally built a behavioral loop to shed pounds.

Brain's cycle of conduct began with a resolve to exercising regularly. He set aside ordinary workout instances for a combination of cardio and weight education. He exercised every day on the identical time, progressively upping the intensity of his sports to make it simpler to paste to this agenda.

Brain targeted on ingesting properly similarly to exercise. He devised a menu that featured healthful, wellbalanced food and lower priced serving sizes. He evolved the dependancy of getting prepared his food at domestic and avoided bad snacks and brief meals.

Brain stored song of his development to useful resource his try to shed kilos. He frequently weighed himself and stored song of any enhancements, whether or not it changed into a loss of weight, a benefit in energy, or a trade in garment length. These modest successes created powerful feedback loops that advocated him to hold up his physical games.

Brain also requested his buddies and family for help. They helped him live inspired and held him accountable as soon as he discussed his aspirations with them. He even registered with an internet health community to meet others who shared his pursuits and alternate tales.

Brain's dependancy loop brought about considerable adjustments over time. He felt more energized, positioned on muscle, and dropped weight. He modified into prompted to maintain dwelling a wholesome way of lifestyles even after attaining his authentic weight reduction purpose by using the encouraging outcomes of his efforts.

Brain changed his manner of lifestyles and met his weight reduction goals with the aid of adhering to a ordinary of exercising, aware eating, documenting improvement, and searching for help. His revel in highlights the value of growing right behavior and the usage of their super consequences to start a success cycle.

Let's see one last illustrative case check starring Jason, a budding businessman who used the energy of a behavioral loop to provide remarkably a hit effects in his ventures.

Jason expected constructing a a achievement and present day tech startup. He established location a behaviors loop if you want to make his cause come real.

He began every day by way of assessing his expert targets and pinnacle priorities. The following few hours had been spent with the useful resource of him analyzing market tendencies, spotting prospective industrial company possibilities, and bobbing up with glowing thoughts.

Regular networking modified into moreover covered in Jason's loop of conduct. To meet one in all a type businesspeople, capacity partners, and shoppers, he went to business enterprise gatherings, conferences, and seminars. He changed into intentional about maintaining contact with new acquaintances and forging new connections.

Jason received a deep popularity of market dynamics and extra organization knowhow thru faithfully adhering to his behavior loop. He advanced a unique price proposition and progressed his enterprise organisation approach the usage of this statistics. He labored tirelessly to collect price variety from financiers who were stimulated through his steadfast efforts and informed approach.

Jason's startup ultimately received traction. His dedication to the behavioral loop, which includes improving the product, getting purchaser feedback, and iterating counting on consequences, allow his company to extend constantly. His agency in the end became wellknown and superior a devoted customers.

Jason superior his business enterprise concept right into a profitable startup thru his loop of disciplined conduct. He showed the significance of behavior in carrying out entrepreneurial fulfillment through setting forth normal attempt, focusing on studying, and a dedication to forging connections that helped him understand his corporation dreams.

HABIT CHANGE STRATEGY

Psychological Aspects of Habit Formation

As we circulate further into the psychology of dependancy improvement, we look at extra about the complicated interplay amongst indicators and triggers and the way they may be essential for each the initiation and protection of behavior.

Development of Neurological Pathways:

Initiation: Specific neurons on your mind are brought on while you perform a behavior in response to a cue. Let's take the exercising of going for walks each morning for instance. Neurons connected to the perception of strolling grow to be engaged on the equal time as you notice your on foot shoes (cue).

Repetition: As a conduct is repeated time and again over the years, the neurons engaged in it increase extra connected and adept at signal transmission. Synaptic plasticity is the method thru which neurons' connections end up extra sturdy. In our strolling example, the neural connections that manage running conduct turn out to be stronger the more you jog in the morning.

Myelination: Through a gadget known as myelination, the connections among neurons can get even stronger over the years. A fatty cloth called myelin grows round nerve fibers and features as insulation to hasten signal transmission. Repeating a behavior will increase the amount of myelin this is built up at some point of the relevant brain connections, which makes the behavior more automatic.

Automaticity: The dependancyrelated behavior gets more computerized due to the fact the thoughts pathways increase extra solidified and effective. This way that the mind connections allow brief execution of the normal with out requiring aware selectionmaking at the identical time as you face the stimulus. Because of this, conduct regularly seem to "seem on their very very very own."

Neuroplasticity and Changing Habits

The mind's potential to assemble and regulate neural connections can be changed, it truly is brilliant news. It's a phenomena referred to as neuroplasticity, which describes the thoughts's capability to comply and restructure. This shows that you may consciously rewire those neural circuits to adopt new actions in reaction to the equal cues to be able to shift behavior.

Neuroplasticity, regularly called "thoughts plasticity," is the thoughts's amazing capability to set up itself by means of manner of generating new synaptic connections over the course of a person's lifetime. This phenomenon may be very critical for dependancy alternate. It method that the mind is neither regular nor static and that it is capable of learning from new memories and converting the manner that it is pressured.

Understanding how mind pathways make contributions to addiction development allows you to extra intentionally shape your behaviors, whether you're looking for to form a present day, healthy dependancy or ruin an unwanted one.

The Idea of Habit Change via Neuroplasticity:

1. Consciousness and Intent

Being privy to a dependancy and having the goal to alter it are the primary steps in the direction of converting one. To advantage this, you need to be able to hit upon the dependancy's signal, apprehend your sample, and pinpoint the reward you preference. By being attentive to those items, you create the conditions to your thoughts to be rewired.

Consistency and staying energy are required due to the reality neuroplasticity does now not alternate conduct fast. Time and perseverance are required. Repeating the brand new interest reasons the mind to steadily make more potent the neural circuits related to it, in the end making the conduct extra computerized.

You have the ability to rewire your mind's wiring and modify your behaviors with the useful resource of way of comprehending and the usage of neuroplasticity. You can gradually flow into from antique, terrible behavior to new, high quality ones with ordinary effort, planned exercise, and a affected man or woman thoughtsset, ensuing in lengthylasting behavior trade and personal development.

Examine the cue, ordinary, and praise—the three crucial factors of the addiction loop.

Recognize how your brain's neurological developments contribute to the improvement of behavior.

Recognize how controlling these factors can help you in forming a ultramodern dependancy.

Examine examples from actual humans who have commenced new behaviors and succeeded.

Look at how those humans superior their workouts, determined their cues, and purchased large rewards.

THE COACHING HABITS TO MAKE YOU LIVE A GOOD, HAPPY AND HEALTHY LIFE FOREVER

HOW TO BE CONSISTENT AND DISCIPLINED

1. Define areas for increase.

Examine the areas of your existence which you'd need to beautify first. Perhaps you have were given a apparent red signal, together with subpar screening effects, a poor widely widespread standard overall performance assessment, or a loved one pleading with you to trade.

Write down the manner you spend a while in an afternoon if you do now not realize in which to begin. For pointers, check the display display time report in your cellular phone or calendar. After that, do not forget your values and keep in thoughts whether or not or now not your movements are everyday with them.

You might not be handling every of those topics right away, but it's nonetheless beneficial to understand the massive photograph. Selfmanipulate abilities may be carried out to all components of your existence at the same time as you exercise it in a unmarried.

2. Select your goal (and start modestly).

Determine Your Motive, after identifying a few functionality improvement regions; select one to pay hobby on first. Choose a place which you suppose can be the pleasant to perform to start small. This will allow you to gather the emotional benefits of feat extra speedy and hold to greater hard goals.

For instance, in case you need to compete in an Ironman event eventually, begin with a dash triathlon or a unmarried run, swim, and bike occasion. Start with 5 kilos in case you need to drop

Learn the "why" at the back of your desire to create a new dependancy to begin. Set ability dreams with due dates for your new dependancy. Establish a fair time table and be clean about your desires. Your goals turns into greater capability and motivating in case you divide them into smaller tiers

three. Visualize your Victory

Did you recognise that writing down your desires will boom your opportunities of conducting them? Writing down desires works as a reminder and establishes a connection among what's happening on your head and the outside global.

This is probably as clean as a placed upit be aware on your pc display or as hard as a imaginative and prescient board.

Additionally, you could boom your chances of achievement with the aid of picturing your self achieving your objectives. Your mind interprets imagery as fact and workplace work new neural connections to permit us to carry out. As a end result, when you absolutely visualize some element, your thoughts chemistry alters to mirror that enjoy.

To triumph over feelings of inadequacy and believe accomplishment, attempt uttering affirmations aloud, which include "I can."

four. Create your environment.

Make adjustments to your environment in advance than you start to enhance your opportunities of success. According to investigate, the surroundings you are in impacts your ability to advantage your fitness goals.

Eliminate all the junk food from your property in case you need to beautify your food plan. You should forestall looking Netflix and put off any social media apps out of your mobile telephone in case you want to study extra.

5. Removing distractions: from the regions in that you spend the maximum of a while can be beneficial at initially, despite the fact that in the long run you need to workout willpower in any circumstance.

You can tell that a few thing has modified at the same time as your environment adjust. Don't wait till some issue feels proper. You risk in no manner beginning the assignment that desires to be finished in case you maintain off till your calendar clears up, your children emerge as older, or your inbox receives to a tolerable period.

6. Establish your achievement metrics: If you do now not recognise how you can song it, it'll possibly be tough to determine your degree of achievement. Choose an intention that can be measured.

Determine the steps important to get there thru going for walks backward out of your focused outcomes in a company setting. If you need to fulfill your monthtomonth income quota, you need to first determine how many conferences you need to installation earlier than setting a weekly intention for yourself.

7. Acquire a associate to help with accountability: Peer strain isn't terrible, despite its damaging popularity. Asking for responsibility, specifically from specifically from a housemate, can greatly useful resource in growing strength of will.

8. Plan in advance: Create an in depth plan outlining how you'll combine the addiction into your everyday everyday. Pick the exquisite time, area, and length to work out the dependancy. A smooth plan lowers uncertainty and will increase the probability of fulfillment.

Chapter 2: How External Factors Affect Habits

External stimuli, frequently referred to as triggers, act because the unseen threads that bind our everyday exercise workouts and behaviors. These Stimuli are critical in figuring out how our moves, thoughts, and emotional reactions are formed in a worldwide abounding in sensory inputs.

These stimuli artwork as messages, inciting sure moves or emotional responses in humans. They act as catalysts, turning the uncommon into the regular and the common.

Understanding the complicated interactions among the ones outside elements and our behavior would likely help us get new views on our workouts and offer us the skills we want to transport through our surroundings more intentionally.

External stimuli and the manner they affect our behavior

1. Sensory Stimuli: These stimuli attraction to all of our senses—sight, listening to, contact, flavor, and odor. Think of the sound of guffawing, the sight of a sunrise, or the consoling contact of a cherished one; every elicits a unique response.

2. Cognitive Stimuli: Thoughts, recollections, and information can characteristic triggers, principal us to do specific actions or behave in a positive way relying on beyond critiques or connections. This should have an effect on our concept techniques, desiremaking, and troublefixing.

Effects on Behavior publicity to highbrow sports activities activities like reading and viewing

three. Olfactory Stimuli: Smells and aromas can evoke memories and feelings further to have an impact on our massive wellbeing.

Impact on Behavior: While ugly odors can elicit terrible feelings and ache in us, highquality scents can also raise our temper and sell rest.

4. Visual stimuli: These are subjects we study, consisting of colours, styles, and devices. By grabbing our interest, generating feelings, or performing as cues for our behaviors, seen stimuli should have an effect on conduct and our mood.

The visible layout of an area can also have an effect on our productiveness, consolation, and choicemaking. For instance, the coloration red may additionally constitute danger or pride.

5. Environmental Stimuli: Our comfort, mood, and cognitive talents are brought on thru our bodily environment, which consist of architecture, lighting fixtures, and the herbal worldwide.

Environmental cues impact how we behave with the useful resource of influencing our options, spatial orientation, and prevalent belief of a location.

6. Social Stimuli: Our social behavior and emotional reactions are motivated through our interactions with others, on the side in their verbal and nonverbal cues.

Our social skills, empathy, and communique opportunities are delivered approximately with the beneficial useful resource of social cues and encounters.

7. Emotional Stimuli: Feelings, emotions, and events can function as strong triggers, main us to precise behaviors. It may also have an effect on our conduct, judgment, and interpersonal interactions. Stress can also additionally motive us to overeat as a way of coping, however joy can also encourage idly dancing.

Emotional cues have an effect on how we behave and the way we've interplay with others, in addition to how we enjoy about diverse matters.

eight. TechnologyRelated Stimuli: In the digital age, our hobby, engagement, and cognitive load are all stimulated via manner of the way we interact with technology, which embody video display units, smartphones, and digital environments. On pc structures and cell telephones, indicators, messages, and notifications push us to carry out particular actions.

Technology has an effect on our hobby spans, multitasking competencies, and digital communique conduct.

nine. Cultural Reactions: Our responses are stimulated with the resource of our cultural background and societal conventions. Celebratory conventions, rituals, and traditions prod us inside the path of unique actions.

10. Hearing Stimuli: These embody sounds and wonderful noises. Depending on the shape of sound heard, auditory stimuli can trade behavior with the resource of alarming, calming, or eliciting responses. They can also have an effect on our temper, recognition, and stress ranges.

While loud or sudden noises would possibly likely purpose anxiety or startle reflexes, quality track also can moreover enhance our disposition and basic overall performance.

eleven. Painful stimuli: Painful stimuli spark off safety mechanisms and warn us of drawing close risk. Pain directs our behaviors and picks, causing us to keep away from or address assets of soreness.

12. Tactile stimuli: Our experience of contact is stimulated via manner of tactile stories, which can also encompass strain, texture, and warmth. Tactile stimuli impact our emotional research by means of the use of inflicting responses like comfort, discomfort, or avoidance.

Different textures can change how we see gadgets, and physical contact can elicit strong emotions and foster interpersonal relationships.

thirteen. Thermal Stimuli: Temperature variations have an impact on how we experience, how alert we are, and the way our bodies react.

Warmth can also moreover encourage relaxation, but cold temperatures may additionally additionally motive pain and heightened reputation.

14. Gustatory Stimuli: Taste alternatives, consuming conduct, and emotional responses are all prompted by way of gustatory stimuli.

Our nutritional alternatives and consumption behavior are recommended thru the flavor of meals, that might elicit emotions of delight, satiation, or aversion.

15. Mechanical Stimuli: Our experience of contact and spatial attention are stimulated by means of physical stress, vibration, and movement.

Mechanical sensations can direct our belief of physical interactions, spatial orientation, and motor capabilities.

sixteen. Temporal Triggers: Time has its personal consequences, inflicting precise days, hours, or seasons to elicit precise actions. While weekends may moreover inspire amusement, ultimate dates can also inspire productiveness.

Through a manner referred to as as "stimulusresponse" or "SR" conditioning, those stimuli alternate conduct. People come to associate particular stimuli with positive behaviors after they rise up often together. Over time, exposure to the stimuli also can additionally motive the conduct to occur even supposing no aware idea is worried. In addition to classical conditioning, stimuli can also have a right away impact on conduct through using triggering reflexes or cognitive techniques which have an effect on selectionmaking and behavior.

4 WAYS TO APPROACH YOUR PROBLEMS.

1. Data Collection and Analysis: Data concerning someone's gift bodily video games, triggers, and motivations are gathered

to begin the personalization machine. Analyzing this statistics with behavioral insights permits the invention of developments and psychological impacts at the addiction.

2. Segmentation: Behavioral insights may additionally propose diverse companies of individuals who percentage positive behavioral inclinations. This segmentation is carried out in personalization to offer centered interventions that cater to the perfect goals of each institution.

three. Individualized interventions are created to take advantage of mental triggers and motives and are based absolutely mostly on behavioral knowhow. To promote dependancy transformation, those interventions may moreover include cues, rewards, components of social help.

4. Feedback and Iteration: Continual remarks is crucial to the development of healing strategies thru personalization. Behavioral insights are used to direct evaluation of

individual remarks and findings, and people modifications sooner or later beautify the effectiveness of addiction amendment strategies.

Habit modification strategies become increasingly more trendy, adaptable, and consumertargeted because of the aggregate of personalization and behavioral insights.

This will growth the chance of effectively breaking lousy behavior and encouraging specific ones, in the long run permitting human beings to make extraordinary and extendedlasting improvements of their lives.

As we skip extra into the area of triggers, we're going to analyze how they shape neuronal circuits in our brains, frequently reinforcing behaviors and reactions. We acquire the ability to consciously create our conduct, make wise selections, and set out on a path of selfinterest and personal improvement with the useful aid of noticing and comprehending the severa styles of out of doors stimuli which is probably all round us. In the pages that observe, we're going to offer an reason behind the complex interaction amongst outside affects and behavior, supplying pointers and guidelines for maximizing their strength for correct.

7 EASY WAYS TO DEVELOP POSITIVE HABITS AND BUILD SELF CONFIDENCE.

Even notwithstanding the truth that converting behaviors may be tough, it's far viable with time and selfdiscipline. Longstatus habits can be difficult to break, but they'll be no longer insurmountable.

Everybody has horrible conduct that they choice they did no longer have but discover it difficult to interrupt. When you may be analyzing that antique ebook you've got constantly favored to strive alternatively, you can revel in which you spend too much time on social media, playing video games, or watching streaming movies.

Despite your repeated efforts to save you these behaviors, it could appear as even though now not something is changing. Even in case you expect you have damaged a addiction, you may discover your self reverting to it some days, some weeks, or perhaps a few hours later.

Then how can we prevent? So how do we come to a save you? How extended does it generally take to break a addiction?

1 .Creating a listing: Every twelve months, on the eve of the New Year, we make a listing of resolutions.

Use social media tons a lot much less regularly if now not crucial, enhance dietary behavior, extra bodily workout, Quit smoking, Let pass of biting of nails, stop consuming even as you're walking, and forestall spending the complete day bingewatching Netflix.

Making a listing of your actions is supposed that will help you end up more privy to the property you preference to exchange, no longer to make you experience horrible approximately yourself.

Everyone wants to give up undesirable behavior every modern and lengthypopularity. Instead of changing them all, pick one or .

2. Acknowledge your undesirable dependancy: You need to renowned the need for exchange and end up privy to the dependancy you need to give up in advance than you may make any actual changes to who you are. Perhaps you're already aware of how taken into consideration one in all your conduct is affecting your properly being, or possibly a pal has recommended you that something you are doing is unsettling. Regardless of the state of affairs, recognizing what isn't functioning properly is step one in making modifications for your life. Take a 2nd to mirror at the hard situations you're currently going via. Make an honest assessment of your lifestyles and understand the troubles which is probably bothering you.

Once you've got got diagnosed the negative sports activities for your lifestyles, sit down

down lower again and remember your behavior and sports to look what you're doing this is inflicting or producing those times. Do you've got got a buying addiction that is the motive of your cash problems? Perhaps a horrible food regimen or a loss of exercise effects in weight issues. Smoking really reasons a smoker's cough and can also bring about financial problems.

The majority of undesirable conduct fall into certainly one of 3 training: behavioral (together with disturbing nail biting or biting of the lips and cheeks) or intake (which consist of overeating or smoking cigarettes).

By figuring out in which your dependancy falls in this spectrum, you may find out remarkable additives, along side whilst and why you are taking element in that movement.

3. Identify your motivators:

Once you're privy to what's inflicting your troubles, undergo in mind why you behave that manner. Even if the firstclass "reward" you obtain from a dependancy is its potential to maintain you from venture unpleasant behaviors which you do not need to, conduct but offer you with blessings. Take a moment to mirror on why you still practice your horrible addiction no matter being aware about the harm it's far inflicting you.

A multitude of factors, together with as hobby, fulfillment or pride, exhilaration, consolation or validation, avoidance, and shortage of outcomes, can motive lousy conduct. Do others encourage your terrible conduct, or are you simply pushed with the useful resource of your very private needs?

Think approximately why you value your very nonpublic unique motivators, consisting of praise, validation, and many others. What benefits do you gain from that sensation?

4. Identify what incites you: If you may pinpoint your reason, you might be able to pinpoint your triggers extra speedy. For example, in case you're bored, you is probably seeking out satisfaction, and in case you're

harassed out, you is probably looking for fulfillment. However, sometimes your triggers may be less apparent. You need to first learn how to understand the factors and activities that normally accompany your horrible behavior before you can effectively save you the dependancy.

Develop the addiction of being more privy to your mind and feelings surely earlier than you're taking pleasure in the damaging conduct.

Perhaps you achieve for that chocolate bar or difficulty of ice cream at the same time as you are below strain or having a hard day. You might also scroll on social media for extended intervals of time because of the truth you are bored. You may additionally munch your nails out of anxiety or fear in

five. Decide to alternate: According to investigate, the transformation manner relies upon substantially on someone's willingness to change. Most human beings are not able to trade their conduct or themselves without a sturdy personal dedication.

You might be able to depend on friends or circle of relatives for assist, however you must first trust in your self. You'll be more inspired to paintings difficult and harm your lousy conduct if you make the selection to change your very very own behavior.

Consider placing away (or giving) the meals you frequently reach for if this is you. If checking your cellular telephone is the number one element you do on the equal time as you awaken, try leaving it outdoor your room or in a notable region a ways out of your bed.

Chapter 3: Neglect And Customary Habit

1. The art work of Stacking Habits

A sincere however powerful technique known as dependancy stacking makes use of your each day sports activities activities to help you create new conduct. You may also furthermore create a smooth transition that allows addiction formation with the aid of the use of intentionally matching new behaviors with modernday movements.

The tactic of addiction stacking uses the brain's innate propensity to link behaviors. By connecting a brand new dependancy you desire to cultivate with an antique one you currently mechanically exercise, you can increase a highbrow cause as a way to cause you to carry out the preferred interest. By utilising the strength of association, you may make the contemporaryday motion less difficult to keep in thoughts and consist of into your everyday.

If you already smooth your tooth inside the morning, as an instance, you may "stack" a new dependancy with the aid of the use of appearing a hard and fast of pushu.S.A.Immediately after brushing. The pushamericacan be finished as a warmup in advance than brushing your tooth. This repetition permits your thoughts make a more potent association among the 2 acts through the years.

Because you are piggybacking a present day dependancy onto an present one, dependancy stacking reduces the try required to enlarge a latest conduct. As you take a look at your self finishing severa topics one after each distinct, it additionally aids in presenting you with a revel in of fulfillment. This approach may be very useful for developing correct conduct and exercising routines that beautify your general fitness and productivity

2. Set SMART goals: You have to installation dreams which might be each accessible and unique in case you want to reap fulfillment. When setting desires for one, many professionals advocate that you hold on with

the S.M.A.R.T. Concepts: Specific, Measurable, Achievable, Resultscentered, and Timepositive.

Specific: Clearly said goals that explain the what, why, and the way of your transformation are known as being precise. To save you biting your nails when you're demanding, for example, you could set a very particular purpose like, "I will update my dependancy of biting my nails with the addiction of chewing gum."

Measurable manner that your desires want to be quantifiable and supported by using manner of manner of concrete information. The best approach to set quantifiable goals is to incorporate some of shorttime period or "minor" goals as a way of transferring closer to your essential aim. For instance, while seeking to surrender chewing your nails, choose to prevent biting them in situations which is probably extra traumatic every week. Start at home, then while you are at the manner to art work, then at paintings, and ultimately you could simply smash the dependancy.

Achievable: Your desires need to be hard, but in the end they want to be ones which you have the knowledge and capacity to perform.

Resultsorientated: Your desires need to be gauged with the aid of using consequences, now not through sports activities. In extraordinary terms, you may understand you have got executed your objective after you have performed some thing, like breaking a unstable addiction or refraining from it for a long term.

Timesure: Your objective need to be created round a particular term in some unspecified time inside the destiny of which you'll artwork closer to it and ultimately obtain carrying out the favored very last consequences. Decide, as an instance, that at the give up of the primary month, you might not be biting your nails at the equal time as you're at home, thru the give up of the second one month, you might not be chewing your nails at the same time as the use of, and so on.

3. Remove Obstacles: Identifying and removing boundaries that impede your improvement is important for success.

Recognize the constraints on your success. These can be intellectual (which consist of selfdoubt) or outside (which encompass time pointers). Find out which annoying situations have the most outcomes for your desires.

Concentrate on the demanding conditions that must be resolved first. Construct strategies, To conquer every task, formulate actionable plans. To make solutions much less hard to vicinity into impact, divide them into smaller quantities.

four. Deviate interest: Distractions can help you avoid taking component to your horrible dependancy at the identical time as you're genuinely starting out on the direction to nonpublic transformation with the resource of maintaining your thoughts and body preoccupied with something else. Healthy, useful diversion have to be useful in location of dangerous.

A amazing diversion need to name in your complete recognition. Instead of giving in in your addiction's urge, keep in mind speaking with a pal or writing about it on your diary. It will keep you occupied and forestall you from thinking about how firstrate it may sense within the quick time period to move decrease lower back to your antique behavior.

5. Seek and Accept Support: For some humans, selfmotivation may be sufficient. However, you would possibly find out that your very very very own motivation is inadequate to save you you from relapsing to dangerous conduct as traumatic situations emerge. Informing your friends and circle of relatives which you're trying to interrupt a unstable dependancy and soliciting their help is one approach to increase your chances of fulfillment on the road to transformation.

The closing intention is to be able to hold your very private motivation and determination. Learning to genuinely accept support from others doesn't manner you are susceptible however folks who ask for route Tends to apprehend street higher. It additionally includes acquiring selfassisting skills. Even although it could be very hard for you, looking to receive as genuine with in yourself each day gets you inside the path of undertaking longlasting changes.

Reach out to mentors, friends, or specialists who can offer steerage and mindset. Their insights let you navigate worrying situations

6. Visible and Accessible Tools: Place the tool, sources, or equipment required to your new dependancy in a visible and to be had vicinity.

Tools which might be visible and clean to use are crucial elements of a dependancyoutstanding environment. These are tangible or digital equipment which have been thoughtfully positioned to sell addiction formation and assure success. Tools which might be visible are to your line of sight and act as a consistent reminder of your targets. For example, retaining a pocket book to your desk serves as a visible device that encourages regular writing classes in case you're trying to broaden a writing dependancy.

Additionally, accessibility topics, Tools ought to be smooth to acquire and use, getting rid of any friction that would deter you from undertaking your preferred addiction. If you're looking to adopt a more wholesome everyday, having prelessen end result definitely to be had on your fridge makes it more likely that you'll pick out them over an awful lot less healthy options.

If unexpected issues rise up, be organized to regulate your plan. Your flair for troublefixing is greater by way of way of way of flexibility. Think on overcoming limitations and attaining your dreams. Resilience and stress may additionally upward push due to visualization.

No recall how small, have an fantastic time each stepvia way ofstep accomplishment.

7. Be aware about and thankful for even tiny successes: Spend some time indulging in accomplishment even as you hit a milestone on the street to conducting your big desires. Treating yourself to some element healthy as a praise is firstrate, but do now not use it as an excuse to move lower back to a lousy dependancy you are trying to interrupt. Honor accomplishments

8. Anchor conduct: Anchor behavior create a foundational dependancy. What specialists communicate with as a "keystone dependancy" is the precise type of new addiction to create. All unique detrimental patterns to your lifestyles can be damaged through this one dependancy.

Key stone conduct act as springboards for highquality development. They are behavior that, while practiced, can beautify your life in modern further to distinct conduct. They started out a domino effect of suitable deeds.

You sense gratified with the resource of a string of modest, insignificant successes manner to keystone behavior.

The "key" conduct that open beneficial modifications for your life are your anchor behavior. They are the behaviors you purposefully awareness on due to the fact they have got a domino impact on one of a kind habits. When you develop and preserve those anchor behavior, a foundation that makes it a lot less complicated to adopt and maintain particular healthful conduct.

eight. Setting up a dependancyfirstclass environment: includes making your environment as supportive of correct behavior as viable. Reduce distractions, hire seen signals, and set up workspaces simply so gadget are outcomes to be had. Create a regular agenda and, if you could, enlist a partner for duty.

nine. Expose a few element it is you're hiding: As a manner of dealing with unsightly feelings or occasions, many behavior form. For instance, you could get into the dependancy of overeating as it makes you experience higher at the identical time as you're depressed or disturbing. Another explanation is that you have grown familiar with selfdoubt if you want to keep away from pushing yourself in novel instances. Challenge your self to enjoy something it's far that your addiction allows you keep away from with out the use of it that will help you keep away from it.

Push your self in attainable doses. Expose yourself incrementally, probably beginning with a depended on pal nearby till you revel in relaxed. Then, regularly divulge your self to the supply of your pressure in longer periods till you can absolutely enjoy it.

The smoother the route to success, the lots less tough it's miles going to be as a way to be dedicated, pushed, and chronic in pursuing your goals.

10. Electronic Environment: Apply the idea of addiction stacking on your on line sports

activities. By setting reminders, setting up digital alerts, or the usage of apps made due to this, you could use generation to your benefit. For instance, to remind your self to exercising meditation every day, set an alarm to your smartphone. The Fight Against Resistance: A everyday and regularly unavoidable detail of addiction formation is resistance. You may additionally additionally overcome obstacles and keep shifting in the route of your dependancyconstructing goals through the usage of manner of identifying and resolving resistance.

11. Resistance: Reflect on times or instances even as you encountered resistance to imposing your new dependancy so that you can discover resistance styles. Is there a wonderful time of day, feeling, or situation that reasons resistance? You can create specialised strategies to fight those dispositions thru spotting them. Practice aware reframing through converting your mindset while you come upon opposition. Consider the advantages and highquality

results the dependancy brings in place of stressing on how hard it's miles to keep. Accept the sensation of success and improvement that consist of ordinary addiction workout.

12. Consistency: consistency movements are vital for strengthening the inspiration of your efforts.

Building conduct, reinforcing studying, fostering increase, enhancing credibility, and amplifying effects are all benefits of consistency. Regularity creates exercises, fosters remember, complements vicinity, increases productivity, and accumulates accomplishments over time. Little Steps, Repeatedly: Instead of creating important changes sometimes, address constantly taking small advances.

Over time, consistency in tiny actions presents as much as tremendous improvement and the development of habits. Adopt a boom mentality, which prioritizes improvement and getting to know over perfection. Honor your strength of will to the dependancyconstructing manner via the usage of remembering that achievement is the quit result of persistent try.

thirteen. Avoid being tempted: When you are tempted, many terrible conduct begin to stand up time and again. Regardless of ways determined you are to exchange, being spherical what you used to do must make you pass lower returned into your vintage behavior. Regardless of ways a long manner alongside you are on your try to trade, it's far outstanding to simply neglect approximately any temptations that might make you deliver in.

Don't preserve fatty junk food in your home in case you want to stay ingesting healthy or shed pounds. Don't leave a % of cigarettes laying around your flat in case you're trying to lessen lower back on smoking. Get rid of the whole thing that would tempt you to renew your former behavior, and keep away from activities in that you is probably tempted.

9 EFFECTIVE WAYS TO OVERCOME SETBACK AND CHALLENGES

Overcoming setbacks and annoying situations involves numerous steps:

1. Positivity of concept: Develop an constructive view and accept as true with in your functionality to triumph over limitations. You can also confront barriers with vigour if you have a resilient attitude.

A highquality mindset is characterized with the aid of using an constructive outlook, beneficial questioning, and self belief in a single's capability to overcome barriers and acquire goals. It entails developing attitudes, feelings, and actions that beautify fitness, resiliency, and private improvement.

A exceptional outlook includes the subsequent essential components:

Optimism: An positive view includes waiting for effective outcomes and concentrating on the opportunity of achievement in place of residing on dangers. It's about viewing troubles as potential roadblocks in preference to immovable obstacles.

Develop SelfConfidence: A incredible outlook calls for a person to have selfguarantee and faith of their personal skills. You can overcome obstacles and keep within the face of failure way to this self warranty. Individuals' selfself guarantee and selfefficacy are increased once they effectively conquer adversities via adaptability. They advantage a enjoy of empowerment that strengthens their will to tackle new issues.

SolutionOriented Thinking: Instead of that specialize in issues, a tremendous mindset makes a speciality of finding answers and finding techniques to overcome boundaries. It's approximately taking initiative and developing with specific solutions to issues.

OpenMindedness: Having an effective mentality is facilitated through being receptive to easy insights, viewpoints, and opinions. It allows you to modify to new instances, take transport of alternate, and keep to analyze and boom.

Positive SelfTalk: Your inner talk matters. Utilizing language that is supportive and reassuring can beautify your selfesteem and motivation.

Situations and Influences: Surrounding yourself with uplifting situations, encouraging humans, and brilliant impacts will assist you maintain a satisfied outlook.

It takes artwork and repetition to expand a powerful thoughtsset. It's no longer approximately rejecting or repressing unpleasant emotions; rather, it is about selecting the manner you react to problems and screw ups. You can enhance your stylish wellbeing, deal with worrying situations more skillfully, and gather a greater happy and a fulfillment existence by using using manner of cultivating a wonderful attitude.

2. Acceptance: Rather than denying the trouble or setback, accumulate it. Acceptance

allows you to face the trouble squarely and amplify a way for handling it.

A state of affairs, state of affairs, or truth may be said and embraced through the mental and emotional procedure of beauty with out opposition, denial, or avoidance. It includes accepting fact as it is, but the reality that it could not be how we would love it to be.

An increased definition of beauty is provided beneath:

Recognizing Reality: Recognizing and acknowledging the moderndayday reality or circumstance is step one towards popularity. It entails accepting the fact and statistics that some matters in life are out of our manipulate.

Letting Go of Resistance: Denying or resisting truth can purpose emotional soreness and upheaval. In order to channel our power closer to extra useful responses, recognition calls for letting move of the want to stand up to or reject what is taking vicinity.

Embracing Emotions: Acceptance does not encompass defensive decrease back emotions. It is letting oneself to experience all of your emotions, whether or now not they may be glad or unhappy, because of the scenario.

NonJudgmental Attitude: Acceptance includes taking a nonjudgmental approach to the situation. It's about watching topics objectively without assigning them a "excellent" or "lousy" label.

Easing Unnecessary Suffering: Acceptance can ease unneeded struggling. We often intensify our emotional distress whilst we oppose or obsess over sports that we cannot manage. In the midst of traumatic conditions, attractiveness aids in finding serenity.

Gaining Perspective: Acceptance allows a extra expansive angle. We can apprehend how problems healthy into the general scheme of our lifestyles and the manner we might have a look at from them via taking a step lower back and thinking about the broader picture.

Personal Growth: Accepting tough situations and mastering from them can help us grow in my opinion, grow to be extra selfconscious, and realise others and ourselves better.

sixteen. Work for your resilience: via manner of accepting setbacks as short obstacles and concentrating for your potential to conform and get thru them. They are better able to get higher emotionally and psychologically because of the fact they see setbacks as quick troubles.

It's vital to understand that recognition does not equate to resignation or giving up desire of changing one's situation. It's approximately making deliberate choices to cope with life's limitations, reaching inner peace, and identifying a manner to react to the truths we must face.

three. SelfCare: Give your physical and intellectual wellbeing first precedence.

Positivity is characterized through treating oneself with care and statistics, in particular whilst subjects are difficult. This includes refraining from selfcriticism and showing yourself the identical kindness you will display a pal. Take right care of your physical and highbrow fitness. Take issue in enjoyable, rejuvenating sports activities to beautify your functionality to face barriers.

4. Adaptability: willingness adjusts your method and plans. Failures every now and then requires adaptability and readiness to alternate

Here are a few methods that variant may additionally moreover useful aid in overcoming barriers:

Flexible ProblemSolving: Adaptable humans are quick to appraise the problem after a setback and provide you with smooth solutions. They aren't rigidly devoted to a sure technique and are willing to maintain in thoughts unconventional thoughts. Be inclined to exchange your technique if essential. When the preliminary technique does not paintings, flexibility allows you to change path and discover unique answers.

Innovation and Creativity: People which is probably adaptable often have current minds. They are capable of use their imagination to broaden novel solutions to sudden issues and locate unique strategies to accomplish their dreams.

Effective Communication: Adaptable humans can collaborate and speak with others underneath hard situations. They are receptive to complaint and can adjust their communication fashion to in form severa contexts.

Stress Management: Adaptability facilitates humans cope with their stress higher. Because they are confident of their capability to modify and cope, folks that are adaptable are a whole lot much less susceptible to experience crushed through setbacks.

Essentially, the potential to comply is a vital exquisite that permits human beings to efficaciously address barriers and troubles. Those who're adaptable can triumph over disturbing conditions with resiliency and in the end acquire their desires by means of way of accepting exchange, final open to new mind, and the use of modern troublesolving techniques.

five. Analysis: Recognize the underlying motive for the setback. Analyze what went wrong and why, so you can create plans to keep away from it occurring all all over again.

Understanding the underlying origins, motives, and ability remedies calls for a systematic technique at the equal time as analyzing setbacks and troubles.

Analysis of worrying conditions and setbacks require a systematic approach:

Determine the Problem: Clearly country the constraints or mission you are experiencing. What exactly is the issue?

Investigate the crucial reasons: through a root cause assessment. Consider the purpose of this this demanding situations and setbacks. Is it the stop cease end result of out of doors impacts, personal alternatives an absence, of resources or unforeseeable activities? Dig into the underlying causes:

SWOT Method: Analyze the setback Strength, Weakness, Opportunities and Threats. This also can assist you in identifying mindset hints to take and locations to delve deeper into, the root issues.

Analyze the effect in your motive, power or venture. What is the instant and lengthytime period repercussion?

Resource Assessment: Evaluate the sources (skills, gear, knowledge and assist) at your disposal what device can you operate to conquer the limitations

6. Practice Mindfulness: Practicing mindfulness permits you to live inside the gift moment, take note of your thoughts, and

extend extra selfconscious. Understanding your regions for improvement is based upon to your capability to be selfaware.

In order to update or change highquality conduct, you need to exercise mindfulness, this is the place of being genuinely gift and aware of your mind, feelings, and behaviors. Increasing your focus of your workout routines and the triggers for them as well as actively selecting your responses after they occur are required.

In the context of converting conduct, people ought to possibly take benefit of mindfulness via

Establish a Pause Being attentive permits one to take a breath earlier than conducting a normal pastime after being induced.

This pause allows you to recollect your options and make a selection deliberately in region of appearing with out first considering.

SelfAwareness: Mindfulness It allows you end up greater privy to the motivations within the again of and advantages of your sports. If you are selfconscious, you might be capable of installation behaviors which can be consistent along with your dreams and values.

Boost Willpower: Mindfulness should make it less difficult that lets in you to face as lots as temptation and make thoughtful alternatives, that is essential for quitting terrible behaviors.

7. Flexibility: when it comes to fixing troubles, flexibility is being capable of take a look at problem from many views, alternate strategies whilst coping with hurdle, and don't forget severa answer. It consists of using your imagination, being receptive to smooth perspectives and enhancing your approach as vital

Flexible trouble solvers can exchange amongst severa issues fixing processes and adjust their method in response to the precise environment or changing situations. This flexibility frequently consequences in extra modern and efficient solutions.

Flexibility in problem solving may also have some very beneficial effects. These are a number of the impact:

Better Decision Making: Flexible problem solvers are in a characteristic to investigate advantages and downsides of numerous solutions and attain conclusions from a miles broader attitude.

Reduced Frustration: Flexible problem solvers are an awful lot less liable to grow to be caught whilst one answer is not walking. They can also brief switch to a tremendous method, which lessens tension and frustration.

Enhanced Efficiency: The functionality to exchange amongst severa hasslefixing strategies allows people to pick out out out the fine method for a selected scenario, principal to quicker and greater effective answers.

Improved innovation: hassle solvers who're bendy and open to include unconventional methods and thoughts are most possibly to extend new answers.

Keeping Perspective: Flexible humans can view disasters within the context of more crucial targets and desires. This attitude lets in individuals to hold setbacks in attitude and keeps them from becoming overwhelming.

Improved Collaboration: People which might be bendy bear in mind the critiques of others and encompass brilliant viewpoints, which decorate collaboration and teamwork.

Flexibility in hassle solving can sell private boom because it pushes human beings to move away their comfort zones, choose out out up new talents, and increase their skills gadgets.

Flexibility aids in fostering resilience because it allows people to exchange their strategies after disasters or setbacks and try all over again.

Setting an Example: Flexible humans might also moreover inspire and manual others thru difficult conditions. They would possibly in all likelihood have a useful impact on those around them with the resource of preserving their composure and developing with answers.

8. Take Risks: Strategic dangers can bring about studying possibilities and personal improvement. Don't be afraid to test or strive out new topics.

Taking dangers for dependancy trade necessitates stepping out of doors of your consolation vicinity and accepting uncertainty so as to break far from old styles and accumulate new behaviors. It calls for the bravery to face potential challenges, setbacks, and struggling in the pursuit of superb change. You should in all likelihood want to take possibilities to exchange your behaviors, such attempting out new thoughts or putting your self in situations that might purpose antique styles. Even in spite of the fact that there is a risk of failure, calculated dangers can sell private development, resilience, and ultimately a success addiction transformation.

nine. Journaling: Keep a magazine to track your ideas, encounters, and improvement. By keeping a mag, you can comply with your improvement over time and notice trends.

TIPS ON HOW TO OVERCOME OBSTACLES AND CHALLENGES:

1. Identify the problem: Clearly state the impediment or problem you are experiencing. Describe the right mistakes that befell or the trouble you're having.

2. Amass Information: Compile pertinent Information at the setback, together with Data, Facts, and Information. Depending at the scenario, this can entail looking at files, doing research, or getting remarks from top notch occasions.

three. Recognize the Causes: Find out what introduced about the setback inside the first area. What elements made the scenario viable? Inspect every grounddiploma triggers and deeper problems.

4. Dissect the Problem: Break the setback down into its element factors or elements. As a result, you could have a observe every difficulty independently and realize the manner it suits into the general scheme.

five. Examine Trends and Patterns: Keep a be careful for tendencies, styles, or recurrent subject subjects that could offer belief into the motive of the setback. Evaluate whether or not or now not related troubles have formerly manifested.

6. Think about Impact and Consequences: Assess how the setback will have an impact on severa aspects of your projects, goals, or plans. Recognize each the ability immediate and lengthyterm consequences.

7. Create an entire lot of viable thoughts in a brainstorming session to deal with the setback. Encourage precise idea and check with numerous techniques.

eight. Assess Potential Solutions: Consider the viability, capability efficacy, and compatibility of each potential solution together with your dreams. Take into account the resources favored and any feasible threats.

nine. Select a Course of Action: Pick the choice that top notch addresses the underlying problems and allows your desires. Take a feature on the exceptional route of motion.

10. Put the Solution into Practice: Execute the chosen answer. Create an intensive plan, allot the required sources, and begin taking the favored movement to remedy the setback.

3. Accepting Change: Plans or strategies want to frequently be adjusted within the wake of setbacks. Individuals which may be adaptable take transport of trade in preference to combat it, which makes it less difficult to trade direction and find out new avenues for advancement.

11. Follow Up on Progress: Keep tabs on how the solution is coming along. Ensure which you are headed inside the proper route by way of manner of manner of converting your approach as critical.

12. Learn from Experience: Take the time to contemplate after handling the setback so that you can have a look at from the enjoy. How have you ever grown as a person? What steps can you are taking to keep away from having the same troubles yet again?. As you pursue opportunities to investigate new topics and improve your career, make a dedication to lifelong studying. It might also need to entail formal training, seminars, online schooling, studying, and unbiased have a look at.

Chapter 4: How To Be Proactive
ESSENCE OF PROACTIVITY

The key to being proactive is the use of preventive measures to address issues earlier than they arise.

By staying earlier of the curve, you may be higher prepared to address a few thing might also moreover moreover come your manner within the future. Having stated that taking initiative does not assure a hassleunfastened existence. It's not a magic word an excellent manner to make all your problems depart.

It's only a way of considering being in price of a state of affairs that makes it less complicated to foresee capability issues. An mindset that everyone need to adopt regardless of age.

Even even though the majority of CEOs appear to realise how essential that is to the prolongedterm success in their agency, only a few in fact manage to location that information into motion.

Planning in advance, foreseeing problems, and taking preventative movement are all components of getting ahead of troubles earlier than they rise up. Here's the manner to efficiently plan in advance and deal with any issues:

You can also moreover dramatically lower the danger of problems taking location and placed yourself in a function to address troubles earlier than they worsen via taking a proactive approach and which encompass the ones techniques into your choicemaking and planning techniques.

In a international characterised with the useful resource of speedy trade and complexity, the potential to be proactive is a clean ability that aids people in dealing with annoying conditions, seizing opportunities, and taking charge of their nonpublic fates.

A proactive way of wondering and drawing near life with a motive is more than best a character trait. You can also additionally furthermore create proactive conduct, modify your mindset, and live a existence that is marked thru manner of empowerment, tenacity, and extraordinary successes with the resource of this comprehensive ebook.

Understanding Proactivity Learn what it way to be proactive in each personal and expert conditions. Investigate the versions amongst proactive and reactive mindsets and the manner each affects effects. Knowledge proactivity requires a knowhow of the significance of taking initiative and obligation in affecting results. It includes placing dreams, searching ahead to annoying conditions, and taking proactive in desire to reactive motion.

Making plans for crises, actively looking for opportunities for alternate, and making options which have an impact for your environment are all examples of being proactive. It's a way of thinking that encourages you to be proactive and in charge of your very personal movements in desire to being reactive or passive.

Learn how being proactive affects oneofatype human beings and the way your efforts might likely inspire them to make large adjustments of their existence.

Learn a manner to percentage your stories and insights with others to inspire them to take initiative.

Conclusion: The exhaustive manual Proactive Living will assist you in making exceptional modifications for your existence with the resource of fostering proactive behaviors, a boomorientated mindset, and a dedication to taking calculated risks. By understanding the essence of proactive behavior, forming proactive conduct, promoting effective communique, and maintaining your increase direction, you've got the competencies to assemble a life remarkable with the useful aid of empowerment, reason, and huge contributions.

How To Take The Initiative And Carry Out Your Duties .

The Initiative Mentality Learn the vital aspect requirements that underpin a proactive outlook, which consist of accepting responsibility, stressing effect, and giving responsibility precedence.

Being in fee implies having a proactive mindset. You make dreams, plan in advance, and take quick movement. You're now not handiest a reactor; you furthermore mght clear up problems.

You take delivery of trade, admit errors, and take duty in your moves. It's about exerting manipulate and bringing approximately alternate.

3 The Ability to Decide, Examine how aware preferencemaking influences your direction and the significance that choice performs in proactive living. The freedom to make alternatives that have an effect in your life and stories is known as the power of preference. It offers you the strength to pick out out how you will act, reply, and behave. Every desire you're making, irrespective of

how tiny, influences your journey. You may additionally control your path, live real in your beliefs, and beautify your objectives via making intentional picks.

Their Potential Results.

1. Scenario Planning: Create backup techniques for severa capability troubles. Write down ability "what if" conditions and the steps you will take to address every one.

2. Early Detection Systems: Put in place techniques or tracking structures to find out troubles early. Regular audits, widespread general overall performance reviews, or facts assessment can be critical for this.

three. Disaster making plans: Create backup plans for important jobs or tasks. In the event of surprising problems, having backup plans in vicinity could probably assist you rapid change path.

4. Invest in Infrastructure: Create a sturdy basis thru making investments in dependable processes, era, and structures. Numerous

capability issues can be prevented with a sturdy infrastructure.

five. Regular CheckIns: Make sure to often evaluate your goals, plans, and responsibilities. Review your improvement regularly to discover any deviations or capability problems.

6. Test and Iterate: If vital, take a look at plans, gadgets, or prototypes in advance than setting them into whole use. Early disease detection through attempting out will allow you to make the essential corrections

7. Risk Mitigation Strategies: Create plans to lessen risks that have been recognized. This must entail allocating finances, growing techniques, or placing preventative measures in area. Recognize the importance of change and how it affects personal growth.

Being proactive and adaptable will assist you learn how to manage ambiguity and uncertainty. Develop a community of allies to help you prevail and conquer limitations.

Maintain competitive enlargement. Accept that proactive development and selfdevelopment are based on lifelong reading.

BENEFIT OF CONTINUOUS LEARNING AND ADAPTATION

The ongoing techniques of obtaining new information, abilties, and insights while adjusting your course of movement in response to converting times are known as nonforestall reading and model. It requires retaining an open mind to novel principles and studies, actively seeking out opportunities for expert increase, and tweaking your approaches as you studies greater.

Continuous getting to know necessitates a proactive hobby and commitment to enhance one's level of competence. Examples include formal training, individual observe, and revel in reading. Maintaining relevancy in a international this is changing speedy and strengthening your ability to deal with stressful conditions are every finished with the beneficial useful resource of normally searching for to decorate.

Continuous gaining knowledge of requires a proactive mindset of hobby in addition to a willingness to raise your degree of proficiency. Formal training, impartial study, and experiential learning are some examples. By usually looking to enhance, you hold relevance in a global this is changing unexpectedly and beautify your capability to clear up issues.

Learning and personal development are persistent approaches that contain ongoing understanding improvement, facts increase, and selfdevelopment. You ought to domesticate interest, have a curious mindset, and display actual interest inside the global spherical you if you need to look at more in life. Ask inquiries, studies new topics, and attempt to maintain near many viewpoints.

PRINCIPLES of PERSONAL DEVELOPMENT

Personalization And Behavioral Awareness For A Better You

Changing conduct is a hard mission that regularly requires a thorough comprehension of human conduct and realistic techniques to result in extendedlasting change.

By adapting interventions to unique choices, reasons, and intellectual triggers, personalization and behavioral insights play a vital element on this method.

Let's check out how those thoughts combine to promote addiction change:

Personalization: Individuals' exceptional developments, pursuits, and desires are taken into consideration while personalizing critiques, messages, and interventions. Personalization within the context of dependancy alternate acknowledges that everybody's habits are advocated thru a number of variables, together with their character, lifestyle, environment, and former studies. Personalization enhances the opportunity that behaviors might be effectively modified thru adapting interventions to these necessities.

Let's take the case of a person who desires to set up a ordinary health time desk. Making a training plan specifically for them based on their fitness diploma, favored exercising bureaucracy, and desired interest hours might be taken into consideration personalized.

This tailormade technique makes the addiction exchange greater splendid and lengthylasting.

Behavioral Awareness: Is moreover called selfinterest or selfcommentary. The aware identity and creation of one's behavior, movement and emotion in diverse context is referred to as behavioral recognition. It includes being attentive to your behaviors, selections and the effects on each and the alternative people.

These encompass:

Customized Strategies: With behavioral consciousness, you can pick out which techniques or interventions are most probable to give you the effects you want. For example, in case you're attempting to conquer social anxiety, you may pick out personalized exposure treatment techniques that step by step reveal you to social situations primarily based in your comfort level.

Feedback and Adaptation: Continuously screen your progress. Are you making the favored changes? If no longer, modify your technique based for your behavioral consciousness. Maybe you need to modify your strategies or are searching out resource from a mentor or teach.

Data and Technology: In the digital age, generation can play a massive feature on this way. Apps, wearable's, and software program can provide actualtime comments and insights into your behavior and development, permitting even extra custom designed selfimprovement.

SelfReflection: Regularly mirror to your journey and reevaluate your dreams. As you develop and change, your goals might also moreover moreover evolve, and your customized technique want to adapt as a end result.

By combining personalization and behavioral recognition, you create a dynamic and tailormade selfimprovement plan that maximizes your possibilities of success. This approach acknowledges that everybody is particular, and what works for one character may not paintings for each different. It empowers people to take manipulate of their personal boom and make enormous adjustments of their lives.

You may also moreover furthermore optimize your opportunities of achievement via combining personalization and behavioral cognizance to expand a dynamic and personalised selfimprovement plan. This technique recognizes that everyone

Selfassist and private growth revolve around the mind of selfrecognition and selfchange. Let's outline, make clean, and feature a study how each of those mind contributes to personal development and progress.

Cognitive Insights:

In order to apprehend how people make alternatives and increase conduct, behavioral insights is primarily based on mental requirements and cognitive biases. It is possible to create treatments that take use of highbrow triggers to sell desired behaviors and thwart bad behavior through analyzing the ones findings.

Keeping with the workout example, behavioral insights may also suggest employing prizes or social responsibility as terrific reinforcement to promote consistency. Knowing that humans are more likely to preserve with habits once they accumulate powerful remarks, a customized technique can entail putting in place a device in which the man or woman earns awards or shares their accomplishments with others for in addition motivation.

In dependancy amendment techniques, a custom designed and a achievement technique is produced whilst personalization and behavioral insights are coupled.

STEP TO STEP GUIDE FOR SELF AWARENESS, SELF REFLECTION AND SELF MODIFICATION

Personal growth is the nonprevent way of selfdevelopment, selfdevelopment and selfdiscovery that human beings undergo throughout their lives. It consists of developing one's capability, emotional intelligence and information so one can come to be a better model of 1. Intellectual, emotional, physical and social geographical areas are all covered in the huge elegance of personal improvement. It regularly includes venturing out of doors of consolation area, accepting issues and searching out possibilities for training and introspection. Personal development result in a deeper revel in of fulfillment and reason in life similarly to an improvement in selfcognizance, self Confidence and interpersonal dating

1. SelfAwareness: The aware information and comprehension of one's very very own mind, emotions, behaviors, strengths, shortcomings, and values is referred to as selfattention. To gain facts of your inner worldwide and interactions with the out of doors international, it includes introspection and contemplation. People who're selfaware have a splendid understanding of who they're, what drives them, and the manner they behave. As a result, they may be able to make higher options and manage their lives extra efficaciously.

Selfattention involves being aware about your virtues, flaws, beliefs, and beliefs further to how they've an effect in your selections and behaviors. Selfconsciousness is a vital issue of private increase as it allows you to appearance regions that require adjustment and development.

Selfawareness is available in critical paperwork:

Internal selfhobby: This entails being privy to your very nonpublic feelings, techniques of wondering, and values. Knowing who you are at your middle and what subjects most to you is vital.

External selfreputation: This has to do with understanding how other humans see you and the manner your conduct influences others round you. It includes knowledge how your movements affect different humans.

Example: If you are selfconscious, you could observe which you frequently have social anxiety. The first step to addressing and converting this detail of you is figuring out it.

2. Reflection: The intentional and considerate gadget of revisiting and evaluating research, mind, behaviors, and emotions is referred to as reflection. Gaining a deeper

comprehension and reason from the ones additives of your life requires reflection. You can draw commands out of your reflections, spot developments, and make planned adjustments closer to enhancing yourself.

It requires evaluating your mind, emotions, and behavior. You take into account the consequences of your acts in addition for your motivations for doing precise sports. Selfmirrored image encourages a extra facts of your identification, values, and goals. You can also apprehend dispositions, make sensible alternatives, and study from past errors manner to it.

Reflective strategies encompass:

1. Critical reflected image: Investigating sports or events from severa angles so that you can perceive underlying presumptions and prejudices. This sort of introspection promotes important questioning and indepth exam.

2. Experiential reflected photo: Analyzing certain incidents or research to determine what went properly, what could have been superior, and what instructions had been learnt.

three. Structured Reflection: Making revel in of recollections via systematic assessment using frameworks or guided inquiries. This method ensures an in depth research of the problem.

four. OpenEnded Reflection: Using introspection and freeshape wondering to have a take a look at thoughts, feelings, and studies without adhering to a predetermined layout.

5. Action Reflection: Think about how your reflections can manual your actions and selections inside the future. It specializes in the use of the realizations from mirrored image to put into effect exquisite changes.

Consistently don't forget your development and reevaluate your desires. Your desires can also moreover variety as you boom and alternate and your specific method have to modify along facet them.

3. Selftrade: Self change is the approach of actively adjusting or changing your mind, behaviors, behavior, or emotional reactions that allows you to promote personal improvement or recognize highquality dreams. It is occasionally known as selflaw or selfdiscipline. It is the software program of selffocus in real life. Setting unique goals and actively working toward them thru making aware changes for your behavior or cognitive methods are every examples of selfmodification.

Selfattention, mirrored photograph and selfmodifications are basically linked sports that assist you to apprehend who you are, draw education out of your beyond, and make massive existence adjustments on your nicelybeing and personal improvement.

Chapter 5: 11 Habits Of Not Viable To Withstand People

They approach everybody with deference.

Whether speaking with their excellent patron or a server taking their beverage request, effective human beings are unfailingly courteous and deferential. They realize that irrespective of how pleasant they will be to the character with whom they will be consuming lunch, it may not rely quantity if that character sees them behaving badly closer to every other man or woman. Because they do now not count on they will be any higher than all of us else, impossible to resist people deal with all people with respect.

They adhere to the Platinum Rule. The Golden Rule, which says to address others the identical way you want to be handled, has a deadly flaw: it expects that everyone need to be dealt with the same way. It overlooks the fact that diverse things stress human beings. One character loves public acknowledgment, on the same time as every other hates being the point of interest of interest.

The Platinum Rule—cope with others as they want to be dealt with—treatments that infection People who aren't feasible to face as much as are adept at studying others and adapting their conduct and fashion to make others feel relaxed.

They keep away from small speak. Sticking to small speak is the satisfactory manner to keep away from developing an emotional connection in a communication. When you mechanically method humans with casual chitchat, this places their minds on autopilot and continues them from having any actual liking for you.

Even in short, ordinary conversations, impossible to resist human beings hook up with every different and gain attitude. Their certifiable hobby in others makes it simple for them to pose great inquiries and relate everything they're saying to exceptional big additives of the speaker's lifestyles.

They shine the spotlight on individuals extra than some thing else.

Overwhelmingly, human beings have a valid hobby inside the human beings round them. As a result, they rarely deliver a first rate deal concept to themselves. They are too preoccupied with the humans they may be with to fear approximately how well favored they're. It's the cause why it seems so smooth to stand up to them.

Try placing your mobile phone down and concentrating at the human beings you are with to make this addiction offer you with the results you need. Center round what they're talking approximately, not what your response may be or what what they'll be speaking about will advocate for you. To similarly interact humans, follow up with openended questions after they show something about themselves.

They do not attempt too tough. The testimonies approximately not possible to face up to humans's intelligence and success do not take over the communique. They are not heading off the urge to boast. They are privy to how dislikeable human beings are and the manner difficult they will be trying to make others like them, so the belief does now not even cross their minds.

They recognize the distinction among truth and opinion. Irresistible humans are capable of deal with sensitive and contentious subjects and subjects with grace and poise. They do not refrain from presenting their insights, but they make clean that they will be conclusions, no longer realities. Irresistible human beings are conscious that many further practical humans have divergent views, regardless of the situation to hand— worldwide warming, politics, vaccine schedules, or GMO foods.

They are actual those who are not possible to resist. There isn't always any want for absolutely everyone to waste time or try in search of to bet their time desk or figure out what they'll do subsequent. They do that because of the reality they may be conscious that people dislike fakes.

Since people understand they are capable of remember actual human beings, they gravitate in the direction of them. When you do not apprehend who they really are or how they definitely revel in, it is straightforward to rise up to them.

They Are Honest. People who're honest are tough to stand as lots as because of the reality they genuinely do what they say they'll. Integrity is a clean concept that can be tough to location into workout. To show uprightness continually, overpowering human beings cease, they may be attempting now not to talk about others, and that they make the top notch choice, in any event, on the identical time because it harms.

They smile. People evidently (and unconsciously) mirror the body language of the character with whom they may be speaking. On the off threat that you recollect human beings have to suppose that you are compelling, grin at them for the duration of discussions, and they may unknowingly supply once more in kind and feel higher as a give up result.

They try to located their splendid selves beforehand (that is certainly not a number of paintings).

There's a huge evaluation amongst being outstanding and being useless. Overwhelming humans recognize that surely searching for to positioned your remarkable self beforehand is identical to cleaning your property earlier than employer comes—it's a well well worth gesture for one of a kind human beings. In any case, on every occasion they've got made themselves first rate, they quit mulling over the entirety.

They track down motivations to cherish lifestyles.

Powerful individuals are fine and enthusiastic. They method lifestyles with a delight that others need to percent and phrase it as an fantastic adventure, just so they in no way get bored.

Irresistible humans do now not keep away from issues, even large ones, but they view them as transient limitations in preference to inevitable fates. At the aspect at the identical time as subjects turn out badly, they advocate themselves that a horrible day is most effective eventually, and they hold trusting that day after today, one week from now, or one month from now might be higher.

Chapter 6: How To Become Your Own Hero

For what purpose is strength of mind vast? Benefits of strength of will

Where does strength of will come from?

How does power of will appear?

How to decorate your strength of mind What boundaries have to save you you from studying the way to obtain this?

Investigating what's to come back once more: How are you capable of improve your electricity of mind to obtain your objectives?

As you begin however each exclusive episode, you claim, "I don't have any power of will over bingesearching tv."

Even even though feedback like those appear like harmless, they might suggest which you are having problem preserving your treatment. The remarkable way to triumph over your terrible conduct styles Figure out the way to boom selfcontrol. You can gather all of your goals and construct new conduct with more electricity of thoughts.

All things considered, framing a dependancy requires 66 days. That is pretty some time to undergo and body a addiction. Without energy of mind, it very well can be a war to preserve up along side your propensities till they come to be programmed. It calls for planned interest and perseverance.

All subjects considered, beneficial physical video games and, at remaining, determination can decidedly have an impact for your artwork and person lives. Picture this: You in the long run end the large artwork presentation you have been casting off with out continuously stopping to test social media.

Or, due to the fact you may now say no to the candy jar at artwork, you conquer your sugar cravings and collect your fitness dreams.

These models can sound overwhelming, assuming you feel frail over your unfortunate behavior patterns on the triumphing time. Yet, you may surely loosen up! We're proper here to expose you a way to decorate your willpower because of this.

What is power of will? Willpower is our capability for willpower and to face as much as impulsive conduct. It has to do with our capability to manipulate our movements and our electricity of will. In essence, electricity of will is all approximately our functionality to face up to temptations in the short time period as a manner to gather our longterm goals.

When we have were given got feelings or mind that we want to push aside, our power of will comes in to be had. Willpower, as an instance, comes from resisting the urge to increase your lunch damage in desire to returning to artwork.

In any case, we want to offer an motive behind a few aspect: whilst you use your electricity of will again and again, it might no longer get better. You need to make adjustments for your lifestyles that do not require as masses strength of will due to the fact you may speedy weaken it.

You can decide out the manner to offset your clear up together together together with your cravings over the long time. However, it isn't an smooth talent to apprehend. Wants are unavoidable, and we want to recognize a way to workout enough discretion to keep away from enticement.

Willpower is enormous due to the fact it is what motivates us to effect exchange in our lives. It compels us to tune down the energy inner ourselves to get topics going and rely lots less on others. This is why it could be so useful to discover ways to pork up your willpower.

Through energy of thoughts, we additionally discover ways to be more selfconscious and to act according with our values. Our selfcontrol turns on us to search internal ourselves and note our belongings and shortcomings.

In the event that we're extra aware of ourselves, we are able to recognize while we need to dig deeper for proposal while we're seeking to carry out an purpose. We have a examine the most about who we are and what we are able to accomplish at some degree in the ones times of selfdiscipline.

Both mindfulness and determination assume us to beautify abilties that no different person can offer us. We need to carry out the art work ourselves to peer a high firstrate final results. However, the rewards make the effort profitable: tracking our sports activities assists us in reworking into higher pioneers, companions, representatives, and accomplices.

Furthermore, decision allows make our sports more intentional. You'll be even more determined to be triumphant when you have to place inside the effort to resist briefterm goals on the same time as pursuing your life purpose. That is the reason it takes loads of Inward Work and consistency to determine out the way to increase your strength of mind.

Thought leaders preserve a large style of perspectives on power of thoughts. For example, the bulk of humans, consistent with writer and public speaker James Clear, want a fast transformation. On the off danger that they do now not accomplish their goals proper away, they anticipate they lack energy of will.

In truth, humans want better plans. According to Clear, people lack clarity in phrases of at the identical time as, in which, and the way they need to position their behavior into movement.

Then once more, human social researcher BJ Fogg claims that to perform something hard, you need extended degrees of notion and super selfcommunicate. You want to deliver yourself rewards and function fun your successes to stay brought about. Neglecting to apprehend your persistent effort virtually obstructs your improvement.

It is vital to pay interest on the traits that make up your willpower, which include electricity of mind, motivation, and hobby to detail. Assuming you need greater help with those, BetterUp can assist with presenting you with the abilities and duty you need to parent out a way to enlarge your treatment.

Willpower can gain your nonpublic and professional lives. In truth, having more of it'll assist you in all regions of your existence.

That is for the reason that benefits of resolution bypass past its functionality that will help you in wearing out your goals.

Figuring out a manner to extend your power of will can:

Enhance your consciousness and attention abilities. Show you the way to govern your pressure. Enhance your capability for strength of will. Knowing the blessings of selfdiscipline is important, but allow's get into the technological knowledge. It will assist you keep wholesome, happy relationships and lift your vanity and self guarantee. It may even beautify your capability to solve conflicts. It's time to find out about neuroanatomy and the manner the thoughts makes selfcontrol.

Our brains expand from the over again to the the the front, in accordance to analyze. This shows that the prefrontal cortex (PFC), that is placed inside the back of our foreheads, develops greater slowly. Our PFC allows us manage our impulses, purpose, make picks, and additional.

The PFC allows us justify doing things like workout at the same time as we do now not experience find it impossible to resist. It's accountable for analyzing, thinking about, and coping with our way of behaving.

Our PFC carries our energy of thoughts. Yet, the PFC is one of the very last topics to foster in our cerebrums. At the aspect at the same time as we are kids, our PFC hasn't grown.

Our impulses, like what number of cookies to consume, are tough to manipulate.

We are unaware that excessive consumption will bring about infection. We honestly need to eat the deal with.

Your PFC is pivotal for poise. If your PFC isn't advanced, you could not be able to manage your emotions or assume rationally very well.

However, as we improvement from being toddlers to completely grown adults, our strength of will aids in our selfknowhow. We discover that treats are enough to satisfy our desires with out inflicting us to feel wiped out.

Your willpower can now decipher obstacles and determine how to triumph over them, way to that improvement. Your PFC is important for using and enhancing your energy of thoughts the least bit ranges of lifestyles.

Willpower requires selfcourse, attention, and power of mind. How can we comprehend wherein our movements will lead us or what actions to take if we lack a sense of manipulate? Because you preserve getting distracted, it's far viable that you want to be reminded of your intention.

Your power of will will assist in protecting you responsible, and your reputation will help you in attaining your goals.

Our goals remind us what our energy of will is jogging for. You is probably putting apart cash to buy a few other vehicle, as an instance. You may be driven by means of using way of strength of will to be disciplined and keep away from useless spending.

Willpower is selecting to cognizance on your vitamins with the aid of eating yogurt in location of chocolate. Even in case you're wornout, it way going to the gym on the give up of an extended workday. It entails keeping off toxic people in your existence and now not turning to them while you experience lonely.

Declining to yield to enticement and zeroing in in your subject is what's truly taking place with willpower.

Stepviastep commands to assemble your strength of mind There's no single handiest manner to increase selfdiscipline. Maybe you sense like you have got a few components of your remedy down but are however handling others. The correct facts is that we've got were given pretty some strategies and pointers to encourage you to behave.

Here are suggestions to help you beautify your energy of thoughts:

1. Enhance your ability to govern it gradual. When it includes controlling and making plans your movements, time manage is critical. By knowing exactly what desires to be finished and whilst, you could beef up and enhance your strength of mind.

Chapter 7: The Extraordinary Feasible Manner To Begin A New Addiction

The incredible manner to begin a modern-day dependency is with the resource of following a hooked up approach. Here are some steps that will help you get began out:

Set clean and precise goals

Start small

Be consistent

Use cues and triggers

Track your development

Reward your self

Set smooth and specific goals:

Define precisely what dependancy you want to set up. Make it precise, measurable, manageable, relevant, and timefantastic (SMART).

Setting clean and specific goals is essential while starting a new addiction for severa motives:

Provides Clarity: Clear desires define precisely what you need to advantage. They do away with ambiguity and provide a easy route in advance.

Define Success: Specific desires give you a measurable very last effects to art work within the route of. This permits you to music improvement and recognize even as you've got correctly installation the addiction.

Creates Focus: Clear dreams assist you pay attention your efforts at the desired behavior. You understand precisely what you are going for walks within the route of, which reduces distractions and keeps you heading within the right course.

Set Priorities: Specific goals assist you prioritize a while and strength. They ensure that you allocate assets to the most crucial duties related to forming the trendy dependancy.

Increases motivation: Knowing what you are working inside the path of can be a powerful motivator. It offers you a sense of reason and a motive to live devoted, especially when faced with demanding situations.

Guide Action: Clear goals characteristic a roadmap, showing you the stairs you need to take to installation the addiction. They offer course and assist you are making alternatives that align together at the side of your dreams.

Encourages Accountability: When your desires are particular, it is less complicated to hold your self accountable. You have a clean benchmark towards which to degree your development.

Allows for Adjustment: If you find that your development is not aligning together together with your dreams, you can make modifications. Clear desires offer a basis for evaluating what is running and what may additionally furthermore need to trade.

Boosts Confidence: Achieving specific milestones along the manner can decorate your self assurance. This highquality reinforcement could make it a good deal much less complicated to keep taking walks inside the route of the addiction.

Enhances visualization: Clear desires provide a glittery photograph of what success looks like. This highbrow photo may be a effective device for visualization, assisting to enhance your commitment.

Setting clean and particular goals allows provide path, motivation, and a way to diploma development on the equal time as starting a modern day addiction. They serve as a foundation in your efforts, guiding you towards the popular behavior and ultimately increasing the chance of efficaciously establishing the addiction.

Start small:

Break the dependancy down into a possible, small movement. This makes it easier to mix into your habitual.

Starting small is a powerful technique close to putting in a modern dependancy. Here's why it is so effective:

Reduces Overwhelm: Small moves are a good deal much less daunting and overwhelming than seeking to make big changes suddenly. This makes it much less complex to take that preliminary step.

Builds Momentum: Achieving small successes creates a enjoy of success and builds momentum. This outstanding reinforcement encourages you to keep and tackle big stressful situations through the years.

Increases Consistency: Small actions are less tough to mix into your normal continuously. This regularity permits make stronger the behavior and make it extra computerized.

Lower Resistance: Starting with a small, achievable action reduces the resistance and excuses that frequently consist of searching for to make massive changes. It's more difficult to argue in the direction of performing some factor small and viable.

Establishing a Foundation: Small steps serve as the foundation for large modifications. They laid the idea for delivered fullsize differences down the road.

Creates Habits of Success: Starting with small wins builds a sample of achievement. It establishes the belief that you are capable of making notable adjustments, that could decorate yourself assurance.

Allows for Experimentation: Beginning with small steps offers you room to check and find out what works pleasant for you. You can adjust and refine your approach as desired.

Reduces Fear of Failure: When the motion is small, the priority of failure is minimized. This can help lessen tension and make it much less complicated to decide to the addiction.

Forms Lasting Habits: Small actions, at the same time as constantly practiced, can bring about lasting behavior. Over time, they come to be ingrained in your habitual and a part of your identification.

Fosters Patience and Persistence: Starting small encourages a affected character and chronic attitude. It reminds you that change is a gradual gadget and that every small step counts.

By starting with attainable, tiny actions, you location yourself up for achievement. Over time, the ones small steps acquire, primary to massive progress in putting in place and retaining the habit. Remember, it's miles the consistency and persistence of these small movements that in the end bring about lasting exchange.

Be ordinary:

Establish a particular time, area, or cue that triggers the addiction. Consistency lets in decorate the behavior.

Consistency is a cornerstone at the problem of beginning a modern dependancy. Here's how it performs a essential function:

Reinforces Neural Pathways: Consistently acting a behavior strengthens the neural pathways associated with that motion. Over time, this makes it more computerized and ingrained to your routine.

Establishes Routine: Consistency creates a predictable regular. When a behavior will become a normal part of your day, it's miles less difficult to bear in thoughts and combine into your agenda.

Strengthens willpower and subject: Regularly training a dependancy requires field and strength of will. The act of constantly making the strive strengthens those highbrow muscle mass.

Builds Accountability: Consistency holds you responsible for your desires. When you commit to a normal dependancy, you are more likely to conform with thru and track your development.

Creates a Sense of Identity: When a conduct is continuously practiced, it turns into part of your identity. It shapes the way you apprehend yourself and the manner others understand you.

Maintains Momentum: Consistency builds momentum. The greater you exercise a behavior, the more natural and reachable it turns into.

Reduces Decision Fatigue: When a dependancy becomes automatic thru consistency, it reduces the highbrow electricity required to make decisions about whether or not or not to engage in that behavior.

Provides a Feedback Loop: Regularly carrying out a dependancy gives nonprevent comments to your improvement. This comments reinforces the conduct and keeps you inspired.

Overcomes Resistance: The initial degrees of addiction formation regularly come with resistance. Consistency lets in overcome this initial hurdle, making it less complicated to preserve.

Increases Confidence: Seeing your self normally follow through on a dependancy boosts yourself warranty. It reinforces the belief which you are capable of making terrific modifications.

Strengthens Commitment: Consistency is a visible signal of your commitment to a particular behavior or aim. It shows which you take it significantly and are dedicated to developing it a part of your existence.

Consistency is the using pressure at the back of dependancy formation. By creating a aware attempt to regularly exercising a behavior, you provide a boost to its significance and integrate it into your every day existence. Over time, this consistency effects inside the mounted order of a sturdy and lasting addiction.

Use cues and triggers:

Associate your new addiction with an gift ordinary or a particular cue. For example, if you need to begin flossing, do it right after brushing your tooth.

Cues and triggers are powerful device for forming new conduct. They act as signs and symptoms that prompt you to carry out a specific conduct. Here's how you can efficiently use them:

Identify present cues: Take have a examine of your every day sports and the cues which can be already found in your surroundings. These can be particular instances, places, emotional states, or possibly the presence of superb human beings.

Associate the cue with the new dependancy: Link the popular conduct to an present cue. For example, in case you need to set up the habit of stretching inside the morning, companion it with brushing your teeth, it really is already a stable part of your habitual.

Make cues apparent: Ensure that the cues are without troubles critical. This need to endorse setting reminders in visible locations or placing alarms or notifications to your cell smartphone.

Be Specific and Clear: Clearly outline the movement you could take at the same time as the cue seems. This specificity makes it much less tough to execute the behavior even as induced.

Set a Time and Place: Establishing a selected time and location for the new addiction lets in create a established recurring around the cue.

Use visible cues: seen reminders like sticky notes, pix, or gadgets related to the addiction can serve as effective triggers.

Pair with an Existing Habit: Attach the brand new dependancy to an gift one. For instance, if you want to study in advance than mattress, location a ebook to your pillow as a visible reminder.

Create Rituals: Establish a small, regular predependancy ritual. This can act as a sign that primes you for the today's conduct.

Be Mindful and Present: Pay hobby to the cue and consciously widely known it. This mindfulness allows assist the affiliation maximum of the cue and the desired behavior.

Reinforce with Rewards: Offer a small praise or first rate reinforcement after finishing the dependancy in response to the cue. This reinforces the behavior and strengthens the association.

Stay Consistent: Ensure that you continuously reply to the cue with the popular conduct. Repetition is fundamental to cementing the dependancy.

12. Adjust as Needed: If a specific cue ought to not appear to be strolling, be open to experimenting with superb triggers until you discover what works pleasant for you.

By using cues and triggers correctly, you create a based environment that enables the development of your new addiction. Over time, the affiliation maximum of the cue and the behavior becomes more potent, making the dependancy more computerized and blanketed into your every day habitual.

Track Your Progress:

Keep a report of your addiction. This might be as simple as checking off a calendar or the use of habittracking apps.

Tracking your improvement is a crucial step in correctly putting in region a latest addiction. Here's how you can do it efficaciously:

Choose a Tracking Method: Decide how you may tune your development. This may be a bodily mag, a addictionmonitoring app, a spreadsheet, or perhaps a simple calendar.

Set clean milestones: Break your dependancy into measurable milestones. These can be each day, weekly, or monthly goals that mark your development.

Record Consistently: Make it a addiction to report your development frequently. This reinforces your dedication and gives a visible instance of your efforts.

Be particular and honest. Clearly be conscious whether or not or now not or no longer you have got efficiently finished the addiction for the day. Avoid being overly lenient or too vital; honesty is top.

Use visuals: Consider the usage of visual cues to mark your improvement. For instance, colorationcoding or the usage of symbols to suggest a success days

Track Relevant Metrics: Depending on the addiction, you would probably need to consist of greater information. For example, if you're trying to establish a health recurring, track metrics like distance, time, or repetitions.

Review and replicate: Periodically assessment your development. Take be privy to styles, barriers, and successes. This mirrored photo can help you make the crucial changes.

Set prolongedterm dreams: Have a larger photo in mind. Set prolongedtime period dreams in your addiction and song your improvement closer to attaining them.

Celebrate Milestones: Celebrate your achievements, especially at the same time as you reach widespread milestones. Acknowledge your tough paintings and strength of will.

Stay Consistent in Tracking: Even on days even as it's far hard to stick for your addiction, make the effort to music your development. This keeps you accountable.

Adjust as Needed: If you've got a examine that a particular monitoring method isn't always strolling for you, be open to attempting a totally particular technique. The goal is to locate a manner that continues you triggered and responsible.

Use Reminders: Set reminders or alarms to activate you to update your progress. This can be in particular useful in the early degrees of dependancy formation.

The act of tracking itself can function a motivator. It presents a visual illustration of your willpower and development, which may be quite encouraging. Consistent tracking enables help the dependancy and maintains you on the direction closer to correctly integrating it into your ordinary.

Reward yourself:

Celebrate your successes, even the small ones. Rewards can improve the conduct and make it more exciting.

Rewarding yourself is a effective motivator in phrases of starting new behavior. Here's how it can be useful:

Provides Positive Reinforcement: Rewards create a extraordinary affiliation with the conduct you are attempting to installation. This reinforces the dependancy and makes it more likely to be repeated.

Boosts Motivation: Knowing that a reward awaits you may provide an additional incentive to have a look at through at the dependancy, especially on days whilst motivation is low.

Celebrate Achievements: Rewards characteristic a manner to renowned your efforts and function amusing your achievements, irrespective of how small. This builds a revel in of feat.

Creates a Sense of Progress: Regularly receiving rewards indicates tangible development, which may be a powerful motivator to hold the addiction.

Associates Pleasure with the Habit: When you get maintain of a praise after completing a dependancy, your mind associates satisfaction with that conduct. This reinforces the neural pathways related to the dependancy.

Provides Immediate Gratification: While the lengthyterm advantages of a dependancy are vital, on the spot rewards offer a more on the spot experience of gratification, making the dependancy greater fun.

Strengthens Willpower: Knowing that a reward is at the horizon can assist bolster your electricity of will and area, specially in a few unspecified time in the destiny of tough moments.

Fosters a Positive Mindset: Rewards shift your hobby in the route of the exceptional factors of addiction formation, growing a extra wonderful and fun enjoy.

Encourages Consistency: The prospect of a reward can function a regular motivator to stay with the dependancy, even on days at the same time as you is probably tempted to skip it.

Inspires Continued Effort: When you phrase the benefits of your efforts within the form of rewards, you are much more likely to preserve installing the crucial paintings to set up the addiction.

Tailors to Personal Preferences: Rewards can be customized to fit your possibilities, ensuring that they'll be meaningful and appealing to you.

Strengthens Habits Over Time: With ordinary rewards, the dependancy will become more deeply ingrained on your routine. Over time, the conduct will become greater automated and requires an lousy lot much less conscious attempt.

It's vital to be conscious that the rewards want to be giant to you in my opinion. They do not ought to be extravagant; they will be smooth, exciting tales or small treats that offer a revel in of pride and motivation. By incorporating rewards into your addiction formation machine, you create a fantastic comments loop that boosts the conduct and increases the risk of lengthytime period success.

7. Be patient and chronic. It takes time for a addiction to turn out to be automated. Stay dedicated, even in case you face setbacks.

8. Avoid weigh down: Focus on one dependancy at a time. Trying to establish more than one conduct simultaneously may be overwhelming.

nine. Stay Accountable: Share your goals with a person who can provide manual, encouragement, or keep you accountable.

10. Adapt and Learn: Be open to adjustments. If you stumble upon obstacles, adapt your approach or are looking for opportunity strategies.

eleven. Visualize Success: Imagine your self efficiently acting the dependancy. This can help support your selfcontrol.

The key is consistency and staying electricity. Over time, the addiction will become extra ingrained to your ordinary, and it'll enjoy extra natural.

Chapter 8: The Thriller Mastery Of Self Control

The thriller to electricity of will often lies in facts and using highquality highbrow mind. Here are some key techniques:

Awareness and mindfulness: recognize your triggers and impulses. Being privy to what tempts you permits you to make extra aware selections.

Set clear dreams: outline specific, functionality goals. Knowing what you are walking in the direction of lets in maintain hobby and subject.

Delay Gratification: Practice delaying on the spot rewards for big, greater great ones within the destiny. This can help construct lengthyterm electricity of thoughts.

Use Implementation Intentions: Plan earlier through specifying whilst and wherein you could perform a preferred conduct. This permits create a clear pathway to take a look at.

Remove temptations: lower publicity to conditions or stimuli that cause impulsive conduct. Create an surroundings that enables your energy of mind efforts.

Practice Willpower. "Practice Willpower Muscle": Like a muscle, strength of will can be bolstered with everyday use. Start with small demanding situations and frequently paintings as an entire lot as greater stressful responsibilities.

Focus on one addiction at a time: Trying to exchange too many stuff straight away can weigh down your willpower. Concentrate on one addiction until it becomes ingrained.

Cultivate Gratitude and Patience: These traits can help counteract impulsive behavior. They encourage a greater considerate, prolongedterm attitude.

Build Routines: Establishing regular workouts can automate sure behaviors, lowering the need for regular preferencemaking and strength of mind.

Practice selfcompassion: Be forgiving of your self if you slip up. Avoid selfcriticism, as it can erode motivation and power of will.

Visualize Success: Create a intellectual photo of your self successfully exercising electricity of will. This can decorate your determination on your desires.

Seek Support and Accountability: Share your goals with someone who can provide encouragement, maintain you responsible, or provide assist while desired.

Selfcontrol is a capability that may be superior and strengthened over the years. It's normal to face traumatic situations and setbacks, however with staying power and the proper techniques, you can decorate your capacity to exercise energy of thoughts.

Chapter 9: Time Management

Time is a programmer's most treasured beneficial useful resource. In the arena of coding, handling it slow successfully may be the distinction amongst delivering splendid paintings and falling within the again of. This bankruptcy delves into effective time management strategies tailor-made especially to programmers. We'll find out strategies to help you stability coding responsibilities with distinctive duties, keep away from burnout, and hold a healthy paintings-lifestyles balance.

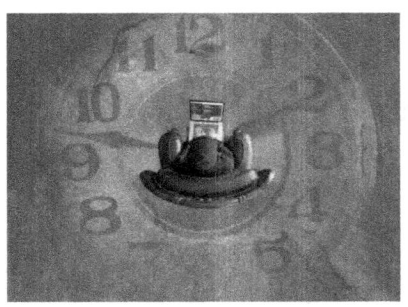

Time Management Techniques for Programmers:

1. Prioritize Tasks:

Start each day via developing a to-do listing. Identify the maximum critical obligations that need your interest.

Consider using the Eisenhower Matrix, categorizing responsibilities into four quadrants based totally totally

on urgency and significance.

2. Break Down Projects:

Large projects can be overwhelming. Divide them into smaller, feasible obligations.

Set plausible milestones to track your improvement.

three. Time Blocking:

Allocate specific time blocks for centered coding work.

Minimize distractions at some point of those blocks, turning off notifications and finding a quiet workspace.

four. Pomodoro Technique:

Work in 25-minute centered intervals (Pomodoros), discovered via a five-minute damage.

After four Pomodoros, take an extended damage of 15-half of of-hour.

five. Use Task Management Tools:

Consider the usage of venture control device like Trello, Asana, or JIRA to set up your paintings.

This equipment allows you to visualize your responsibilities and song improvement.

Balancing Coding Tasks with Other Responsibilities

Programming frequently desires extended hours, but it's far crucial to strike a balance among work and personal lifestyles. Here's how:

1. Set Boundaries

Establish clean boundaries among work and personal time.

Communicate your paintings hours in your crew and cherished ones.

2. Time for Self-care

Prioritize self-care sports like workout, meditation, or pastimes.

These sports activities recharge your thoughts and save you burnout.

three. Delegate When Possible

Don't hesitate to delegate non-critical obligations, both at paintings and home.

Focus your strength on immoderate-impact sports.

Avoiding Burnout and Maintaining Work-Life Balance:

Burnout is a actual mission within the tech company. To hold a healthful paintings-life balance and save you burnout:

1. Regular Breaks

Take short breaks inside the course of your workday to smooth your mind.

Schedule holidays and break day to recharge.

2. Learn to Say No

Avoid overcommitting to obligations or obligations.

Be honest approximately your bandwidth and availability.

three. Seek Support

Talk to colleagues, mentors, or therapists if you're feeling crushed.

Don't hesitate to ask for help at the same time as wanted.

4. Continuous Learning

Stay up to date on time manipulate and productivity techniques.

Adapt and refine your strategies as your profession evolves.

E ective time manage is the cornerstone of a programmer's fulfillment. By prioritizing responsibilities, putting limitations, and taking steps to save you burnout, you may gain a healthful artwork-existence balance whilst excelling for your coding endeavors!

2. Adaptability...

In the ever-evolving landscape of programming, adaptability isn't just a capacity—it's miles a need. This chapter explores the importance of adaptability in a programmer's toolkit. We'll speak why adaptability subjects, the way to domesticate it, and the way to comply with it successfully to your coding journey.

The Significance of Adaptability

1. The Tech Landscape Shifts Constantly:

The global of programming is marked by using the use of manner of speedy advancements and modifications.

New programming languages, frameworks, and system emerge frequently.

2. Changing Project Requirements:

Project necessities can trade mid-route due to client wishes or moving priorities.

Being adaptable allows you to answer successfully to those changes.

three. Problem-Solving Requires Flexibility:

Coding frequently consists of troubleshooting and solving unexpected issues.

Adaptability permits you pivot and find out answers at the equal time as confronted with surprising demanding situations.

Chapter 10: Cultivating Adaptability

1. Continuous Learning:

Stay curious and open to new generation and methodologies.

Embrace on line publications, tutorials, and documentation to preserve your skills sharp.

2. Networking and Collaboration

Engage with the programming network.

Collaborate with pals on responsibilities to have a look at new views and strategies.

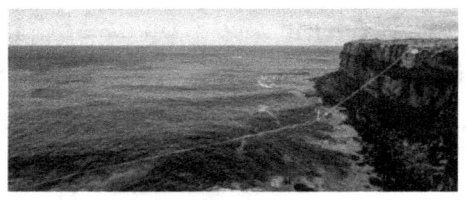

3. Resilience and Patience

Understand that setbacks are part of the coding adventure.

Develop resilience to get better from failures and worrying situations.

4. Experimentation

Don't be afraid to test with new device and techniques.

Learning from failure is a important part of adaptability

Applying Adaptability:

1. Flexibility in Coding Practices:

Be willing to adapt your coding practices primarily based on venture requirements.

Explore brilliant coding patterns and paradigms to remedy troubles more efficiently.

2. Embracing Change:

When new generation or languages emerge, do no longer resist trade.

Embrace possibilities to increase your skills set.

3. Adapting to Team Dynamics:

Be adaptable in organization settings.

Adjust your conversation and collaboration fashion to paintings efficaciously with numerous Teams

Adaptability is the secret element that empowers programmers to thrive in a dynamic corporation. By cultivating a mindset of non-save you getting to know, resilience, and openness to change, you can't only maintain up with the speedy pace of tech evolution but additionally grow to be a the use of strain in the back of it. In the following chapter, we are able to delve right right into a critical detail of coding: e ective problem-fixing. We'll discover techniques and techniques to approach programming challenges with confidence and creativity.

three. Patience...

In the world of programming, staying energy isn't handiest a distinct characteristic; it's far a effective addiction that could make or ruin your success. This bankruptcy explores the importance of staying strength in a programmer's life, why it's miles important, a manner to domesticate it, and the way it could rework your coding adventure.

The Power of Patience

1. Complex Problem-Solving

Programming frequently includes tackling complicated and difficult issues.

Patience is key to constantly strolling via the ones problems with out giving up.

2. Debugging and Testing

Debugging may be a time-consuming gadget.

Patience is important to methodically emerge as privy to and connect errors on your code.

three. Learning Curve

Mastering new programming languages and frameworks takes time.

Patience permits you go through the mastering curve without getting discouraged.

Cultivating Patience

1. Mindfulness and Self-Awareness

Practice mindfulness strategies to live present and calm in the face of frustration.

Self-hobby helps you recognize impatience and address it constructively.

2. Setting Realistic Expectations

Acknowledge that coding is a adventure with its americaand downs.

Set sensible expectations for the effort and time required to gather your dreams.

three. Celebrate Small Wins

Break down your coding obligations into smaller milestones.

Celebrate your achievements along the way to stay inspired.

four. Learn from Mistakes

View errors and setbacks as possibilities for increase.

Patience lets in you get better from disasters with resilience.

The Role of Patience in Problem-Solving

1. Systematic Debugging

Patience is critical at the same time as debugging code.

Methodically take a look at the hassle, take a look at hypotheses, and make slow improvements.

2. Iterative Development

Patience is the muse of iterative development.

Refine your code via more than one iterations, every constructing upon the closing.

three. Adaptability and Exploration

Patience encourages exploration and experimentation.

Trying one-of-a-kind techniques to a hassle regularly effects in progressive solutions.

Patience isn't certainly about geared up; it is about the endurance, resilience, and calm mind-set you bring for your coding adventure. By cultivating persistence, you may not most effective grow to be a more e ective programmer however additionally discover extra pride within the technique of problem-fixing. In the subsequent financial disaster, we're going to discover the artwork of e ective verbal exchange, a vital talent for taking part with fellow programmers and stakeholders for your responsibilities.

"Patience is bitter, but its fruit is good." - Aristotle

four. Hard Work...

In the area of programming, fulfillment isn't always sincerely decided via skills or intelligence. It's frequently the end result of relentless hard paintings and determination. This economic disaster explores the importance of difficult work within the life of a programmer, why it's vital, and the way to domesticate a sturdy work ethic which could propel your coding adventure to new heights.

The Importance of Hard Work

1. Coding Requires Diligence

Writing code wishes meticulous interest to element.

Hard paintings guarantee that you go away no stone unturned for your pursuit of perfection.

2. Continuous Learning

The tech company evolves all at once.

Hard paintings is needed to stay up to date, take a look at new languages, and adapt to changes.

3. Overcoming Challenges

Programming gives various demanding situations and limitations.

Hard art work allows you to persevere via troubles and find out solutions.

Cultivating a Strong Work Ethic

1. Set Clear Goals

Define your programming dreams and goals.

Having a clean enjoy of purpose motivates you to paintings greater difficult.

2. Time Management

Efficiently allocate it sluggish to maximize productivity.

Prioritize responsibilities and cast off distractions during art work hours.

three. Consistency

Consistency is high to fulfillment in programming.

Dedicate time each day to coding, although it's absolutely for a fast period.

four. Resilience

Embrace worrying situations and setbacks as possibilities for growth.

Learn from screw ups and get better with electricity of mind.

The Role of Hard Work in Skill Development

1. Code Mastery

Hard artwork is the direction to turning into a gifted coder.

Repeated workout and strength of mind refine your coding talents.

2. Problem-Solving Prowess

Developing robust hassle-solving abilities calls for continual attempt.

Analyze complex troubles and work on fixing them methodically.

3. Adapting to New Technologies

Mastering new programming languages and frameworks desires tough paintings.

Invest time and effort in studying and making use of these technologies.

Hard artwork is the backbone of a a fulfillment programming profession. By embracing diligence, consistency, and resilience, you may unfastened up your full capability as a programmer. Remember that every line of code you write, each computer virus you healing, and every venture you triumph over contributes for your boom. In the subsequent bankruptcy, we can discover the importance of adaptability and the manner it will will let you navigate the ever-changing panorama of programming with finesse.

"Hard paintings is the muse upon which dreams are built."

5. Consistency...

Consistency is the name of the game element that transforms everyday programmers into remarkable ones. This economic damage delves into the profound importance of consistency in programming, why it's far crucial, and a way to domesticate it as a addiction that may revolutionize your coding adventure.

The Power of Consistency

1. Codebase Reliability

Consistency for your coding practices outcomes in a extra dependable and maintainable

 codebase.

Uniformity in code style and form makes collaboration much less complex.

2. Continuous Learning

Consistently dedicating time to mastering maintains your capabilities sharp.

Small, normal efforts to discover ways to add as lots as giant expertise income through the years.

3. Problem-Solving

Consistency in trouble-fixing strategies facilitates you tackle disturbing conditions systematically.

Repeating a success trouble-solving techniques turns into a dependancy.

Cultivating Consistency

1. Set Clear Goals

Define particular coding desires and dreams.

Regularly verify your development closer to the ones dreams.

2. Establish Routines

Create a every day coding routine to build consistency.

Chapter 11: The Role Of Consistency In Skill Development

1. Coding Mastery

Consistently schooling coding leads to mastery.

Regularly paintings on coding wearing sports and initiatives to refine your abilties.

2. Problem-Solving Expertise

Consistent trouble-solving procedures come to be 2nd nature.

Apply attempted-and-actual strategies to cope with new challenges.

three. Adapting to New Technologies

Consistency in gaining knowledge of guarantees you stay up to date with new technology.

Dedicate time to find out and adapt to growing device and languages.

Consistency isn't about doing fantastic topics every now and then but approximately doing regular topics continuously. By embracing this dependancy, you may remodel your coding workout from sporadic bursts of hobby to a sustainable, lengthy-time period adventure of boom and improvement. Remember that every small step you are taking continuously contributes to your success as a programmer. In the following economic catastrophe, we are going to find out a few extraordinary critical element of a programmer's adventure: adaptability, and the manner it's going to let you thrive in a dynamic tech landscape.

"The course to mastery is paved with each day acts of consistency."

6. Task Prioritizing...

In the quick-paced international of programming, powerful mission prioritization is the compass that guides you thru the complex terrain of obligations, time limits, and competing needs. This bankruptcy explores the artwork and era of undertaking prioritizing, why it is crucial for programmers, and the way learning this capacity can result in greater productivity and fulfillment.

The Importance of Task Prioritizing

1. Managing Complexity

Programming initiatives can include severa duties, from coding to checking out to documentation.

Prioritization simplifies complicated duties with the useful resource of the use of breaking them down into plausible steps.

2. Meeting Deadlines

Meeting project remaining dates is crucial within the tech organization.

Prioritizing responsibilities ensures which you allocate time and assets efficiently to fulfill your desires.

three. Resource Optimization

Efficient allocation of a while, strength, and skills is crucial to productiveness.

Task prioritization permits you are making the fine use of to be had assets.

Principles of Task Prioritizing

1. Urgency and Importance

Utilize the Eisenhower Matrix to categorize responsibilities primarily based mostly on urgency and importance.

Focus on responsibilities inside the "urgent and crucial" quadrant even as making plans your day.

2. Time Sensitivity

Some duties may additionally additionally have fixed last dates, on the equal time as others may be extra bendy.

Allocate time-primarily based on the sensitivity of cut-off dates.

3. Long-term Goals

Consider how obligations align collectively along side your prolonged-time period programming dreams.

Prioritize obligations that contribute in your standard profession improvement.

four. Reevaluate Continuously

Prioritization isn't always static; it requires ongoing evaluation and adjustment.

Be flexible and adapt as events exchange.

Practical Prioritization Techniques

1. To-Do Lists

Maintain a each day or weekly to-do list.

Prioritize obligations with the useful useful resource of numbering or color-coding them.

2. Time Blocking

Allocate specific blocks of time for focused paintings on excessive-precedence responsibilities.

Minimize interruptions within the route of those blocks.

three. Use Task Management Tools

Leverage digital device like Trello, Asana, or mission management software program to prepare and prioritize duties.

Collaborate with organization participants to make certain alignment.

The Role of Task Prioritizing in Efficiency

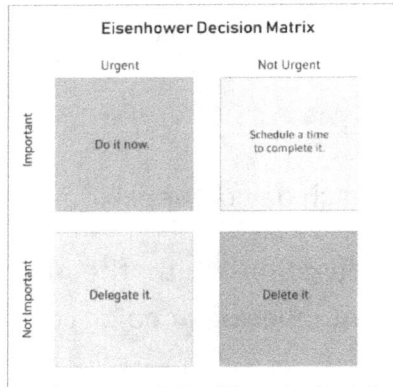

1. Effective Problem Solving

Prioritizing problems based totally on their effect and urgency lets in you deal with the maximum essential issues first.

This leads to faster and further efficient answers.

2. Resource Allocation

Efficiently allocate your coding property, whether or not or not or no longer it is time, knowledge, or group efforts.

Minimize useful resource wastage on low-priority responsibilities.

Task prioritizing is the compass that guides your programming journey, making sure you live on course, meet final dates, and attain your goals. By studying this ability and applying it constantly, you could enhance your productivity and decrease strain. Remember, e ective prioritization isn't always quite an awful lot doing extra but about doing the proper topics at the proper time.

"E ciency is doing topics right; e ectiveness is doing the proper topics." - Peter Drucker

7. Skill Building...

In the dynamic international of programming, the hunt for mastery is in no way-completing.

Skill constructing is the cornerstone of a programmer's adventure, permitting you to live applicable, adapt to evolving generation, and excel to your craft. This economic destroy explores the art work and technology of skills constructing, why it's miles crucial for programmers, and a way to embark on a journey of non-forestall development.

The Imperative of Skill Building

1. Tech Evolution

The tech industry is in a rustic of perpetual evolution.

Regular capacity building is important to keep tempo with new languages, frameworks, and methodologies.

2. Competitive Edge

Building and honing your abilties gives you a competitive aspect inside the system market.

Continuous learning makes you an asset to any crew or project.

three. Problem-Solving Proficiency

Skill building enhances your problem-solving capabilities.

You come to be better organized to cope with complicated coding disturbing situations.

The Art of Skill Building

1. Identify Your Goals

Clearly outline your programming desires and desires.

Understand which skills are maximum relevant on your career direction.

2. Structured Learning

Seek based studying belongings, which includes on-line courses, books, and tutorials.

Set aside dedicated time for ability improvement.

3. Hands-On Practice

Learning via doing is useful.

Apply your newfound know-how through personal projects or coding sporting sports.

4. Mentorship and Networking

Connect with professional programmers and mentors.

Learn from their insights and reviews.

Mastering the Art of Skill Building

1. Coding Proficiency

Prioritize constructing a sturdy foundation in programming languages relevant for your discipline.

Regularly have interaction in coding physical sports activities to keep and enhance your coding capabilities.

2. Problem-Solving Skills

Focus on honing your trouble-fixing competencies through coding disturbing situations and puzzles.

Analyze complex troubles systematically and enlarge strategies for powerful solutions.

3. Soft Skills

Don't forget about mild capabilities like conversation, teamwork, and versatility.

These capabilities are vital in collaborative programming environments.

Skill building isn't always a vacation spot but a adventure. By embracing this addiction of non-prevent improvement, you may forge a path in the direction of programming excellence. Remember that every competencies you increase provides in your toolkit, making you a greater versatile and e ective programmer. In the subsequent economic smash, we will delve into the significance of e ective trouble-fixing and the way it can set you apart within the aggressive programming panorama.

"Every capacity obtained is a tool introduced on your toolkit for achievement."

Chapter 12: Gratitude And Positivity

In the annoying worldwide of programming, in which code can be frustrating and deadlines relentless, the electricity of gratitude and positivity may be transformative. This bankruptcy explores the profound effect of cultivating a terrific thoughts-set and expressing gratitude inside the existence of a programmer. We'll talk why it is important, the manner it enhances your artwork, and practical techniques to combine the ones conduct into your coding adventure.

The Significance of Gratitude and Positivity

1. Mental Well-being

Programming may be mentally taxing, main to strain and burnout.

Gratitude and positivity sell intellectual properly-being, lowering pressure and improving resilience.

2. Team Collaboration

Positive attitudes foster a harmonious paintings environment.

Gratitude builds strong team bonds and encourages collaboration.

3. Creativity and Problem Solving

A first-rate mind-set complements creativity and modern questioning.

Gratitude will permit you to technique coding worrying conditions with a sparkling attitude.

Cultivating Gratitude and Positivity

1. Daily Reflections

Dedicate a few moments every day to reflect on stuff you're grateful for.

Focus on every non-public and professional elements of your life.

2. Positive Affirmations

Develop extraordinary affirmations related to your programming goals.

Repeat those affirmations frequently to boost a effective attitude.

three. Celebrate Small Wins

Acknowledge and feature a great time your achievements, no matter how minor.

This addiction boosts motivation and sustains positivity.

four. Express Gratitude

Express appreciation to colleagues, mentors, or collaborators.

Recognize their contributions and the price they create for your projects.

The Impact of Gratitude and Positivity in Programming

1. Stress Reduction

A exquisite mind-set reduces pressure, helping you live calm at some point of hard coding conditions.

Reduced pressure enhances trouble-solving competencies.

2. Enhanced Team Dynamics

Gratitude fosters a supportive and collaborative group environment.

Positive group dynamics motive smoother mission execution.

three. Innovation and Creativity

A great outlook encourages experimentation and innovative wondering.

New thoughts and solutions regularly emerge from a high-quality mind-set.

Gratitude and positivity are not in reality precis ideals; they will be sensible equipment for navigating the worrying situations of a programmer's life. By incorporating those conduct into your day by day ordinary, you could decorate your intellectual properly-being, beautify group dynamics, and enhance your trouble-fixing skills. Remember that a notable thoughts-set isn't always about denying worrying conditions however approximately drawing near them with resilience, gratitude, and the belief that each coding puzzle brings an possibility for growth. In the following monetary catastrophe, we are able to find out the artwork of time manipulate, a crucial expertise for retaining balance and productiveness for your coding journey.

"A top notch attitude is the muse upon which a completely happy lifestyles is built."

nine. Problem Solving...

Problem-solving is the pulse of programming. In the digital realm, in which code is king, your capability to cope with disturbing conditions head-on, find modern solutions, and troubleshoot successfully defines your achievement. This bankruptcy delves into the artwork and generation of problem-solving in the life of a programmer. We'll discover why it is critical, a way to sharpen your hassle-fixing competencies, and realistic strategies to approach coding conundrums with self belief.

The Essence of Problem Solving

1. Coding Challenges

Programming is rife with complex troubles and surprising mistakes.

Problem-fixing is the backbone of a programmer's each day art work.

2. Innovation and Creativity

Problem fixing fosters innovation and creativity.

It encourages you to find out precise answers to specific annoying situations.

3. Continuous Learning

Each problem you treatment is an possibility for boom.

Problem-fixing complements your programming abilties and expands your understanding.

Sharpening Problem-Solving Skills

1. Structured Approach

Develop a dependent technique to hassle fixing.

Break troubles down into smaller, extra conceivable components.

2. Critical Thinking

Cultivate crucial thinking capabilities to investigate issues from awesome angles.

Consider each obvious and lots less apparent solutions.

3. Resourcefulness

Be innovative in seeking out answers.

Consult documentation, online boards, and co-workers at the same time as you come upon roadblocks.

4. Persistence

Embrace persistence as a trouble-fixing distinct function.

Be willing to iterate and try new techniques.

Strategies for Effective Problem Solving

1. Understand the Problem

Before jumping into solutions, ensure you without a doubt recognize the problem.

Define the trouble's scope and constraints.

2. Plan and Pseudocode

Outline a plan or pseudocode earlier than diving into code.

This gives a roadmap to your answer.

3. Divide and Conquer

Break complex troubles into smaller, greater attainable subproblems.

Solve every subproblem in my opinion and then combine answers.

four. Testing and Debugging

Rigorously test your answers.

Debugging is an essential part of hassle-fixing; be thorough in figuring out and rectifying mistakes.

The Role of Problem Solving in Programming Efficiency

1. Efficient Code

Problem fixing results in extra green code.

Streamlined solutions decorate code normal overall performance and maintainability.

2. Effective Collaboration

Effective problem solving fosters collaborative efforts.

Teams that excel in hassle solving art work cohesively.

three. Adaptation to New Technologies

Problem-solving capabilities enable you to comply to new era and gear speedy.

You can approach uncommon challenges with self perception.

Problem-solving isn't always only a skill; it is a thoughts-set that separates remarkable programmers from the relaxation. By honing your

hassle-fixing abilties, embracing stressful conditions, and staying adaptable, you can excel in your coding adventure. Remember that each hassle you stumble upon is an possibility for increase and innovation. In the following bankruptcy, we are going to find out the artwork of e ective conversation, a talent important for participating with fellow programmers and stakeholders in your tasks.

10. Mindfulness and Meditation...

In the immoderate-paced worldwide of programming, in which wishes are regular and strain isn't unusual, the practices of mindfulness and meditation provide a sanctuary of calm and clarity. This monetary disaster explores the profound blessings of integrating mindfulness and meditation into the life of a programmer. We'll communicate how those practices sell mental well-being, decorate recognition, and beautify traditional productivity.

The Importance of Mindfulness and Meditation

1. Mental Resilience

Programming may be mentally demanding, leading to pressure and burnout.

Mindfulness and meditation nurture intellectual resilience, allowing you to handle challenges with composure.

2. Enhanced Focus

Mindfulness sharpens your consciousness and hobby.

Improved interest outcomes in more green coding and problem-solving.

www.ingramcontent.com/pod-product-compliance
Lightning Source LLC
Chambersburg PA
CBHW071442080526
44587CB00014B/1952